TBI HOPE Magazine
Photography
Contest

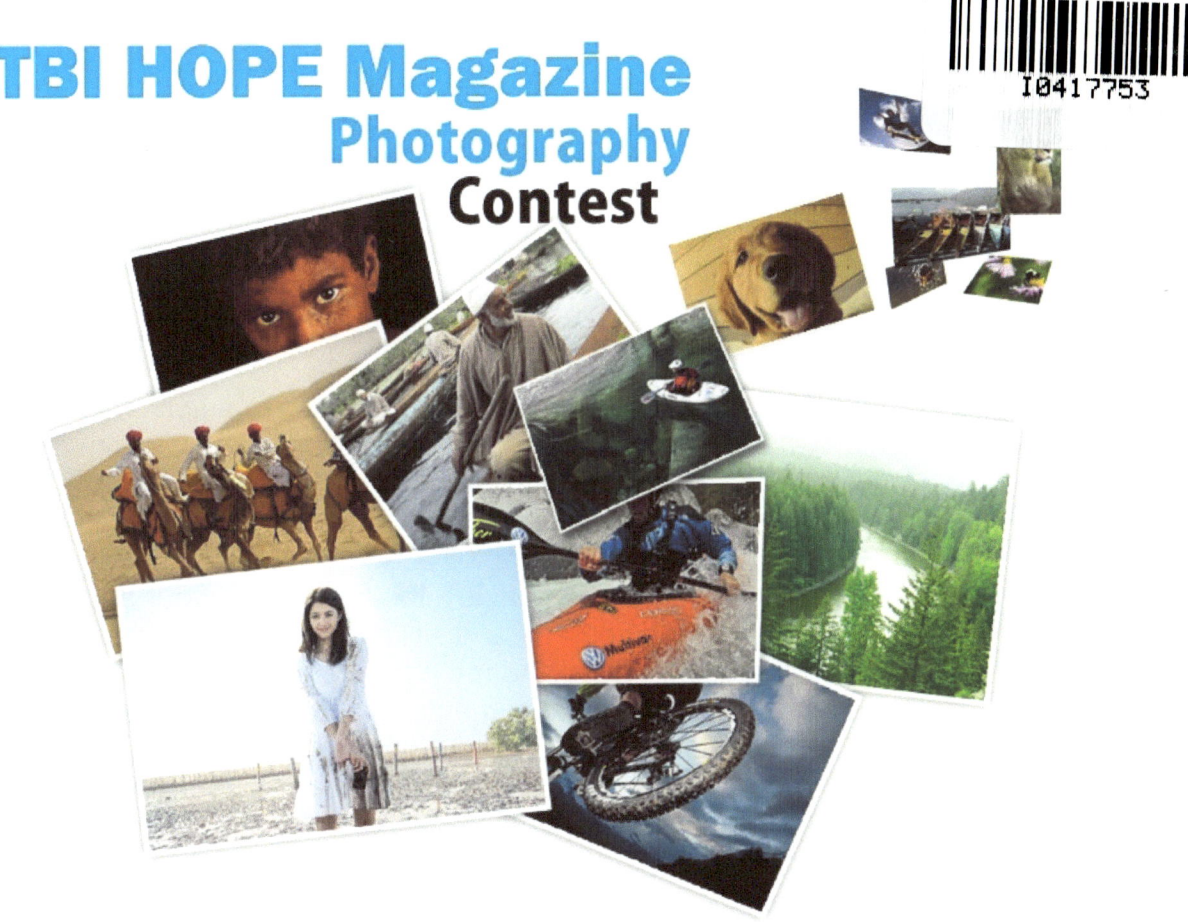

Enter to Win

We are pleased to present our second annual reader photo contest!

Send us your BEST SHOT

We'd love to see pictures of you fully engaged in life as a survivor, though any photo will be considered.

Winners will be published in next month's issue.

There Will Be Prizes!

Winners will receive a printed copy of TBI HOPE Magazine that includes the winning photos

Email your photo submission to photos@tbihopeandinspiration.com.

Submission deadline is 7/25/2017. One entry per reader.
Copyright protected images will not be accepted.

Welcome

TBI HOPE MAGAZINE

Serving All Impacted by Brain Injury

July 2017

Publisher
David A. Grant

Editor
Sarah Grant

Contributing Writers
Janet M. Cromer
Jen Dodge
Donna O'Donnell Figurski
David A. Grant
Rosalie Johnson
Jim Martin
Derek O'Brien
Melissa Robison
Barbara Webster
Amy Zellmer

Amazing Cartoonist
Patrick Brigham

FREE subscriptions at
www.TBIHopeMagazine.com

Welcome to the July 2017 issue of TBI HOPE Magazine!

Again this month, we bring you stories of survivors and those who love them. To our new readers, a warm welcome. TBI HOPE Magazine is the largest and fastest growing magazine serving the brain injury community.

Our contributing writers are the heartbeat of our publication. Without their courage and willingness to share, there would be no publication. I marvel at the perseverance shared in the telling of their stories. Month by month, as my wife Sarah and I review story submissions, we are again reminded that with love, support, and encouragement, lives can indeed be rebuilt in spite of seemingly insurmountable odds.

I want to offer a special shout-out to first-time contributor Derek O'Brien. Back in 2005, Derek not only sustained a brain injury, but was also paralyzed from diving headfirst into a sandbar. As his story shows, attitude really is everything. Derek, you have my respect and admiration for all that you have accomplished.

Every story has value. If you would like to consider sharing yours, I'd love to hear from you. You can email me personally at david@tbihopeandinspiration.com.

Peace,

David A. Grant
Publisher

Contents

What's Inside

July 2017

*TBI HOPE Magazine - Serving Readers
in Over Thirty-Five Countries Around the Globe!*

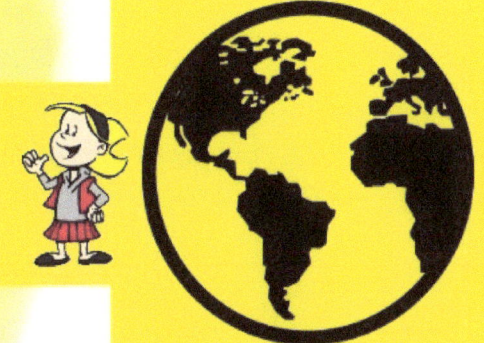

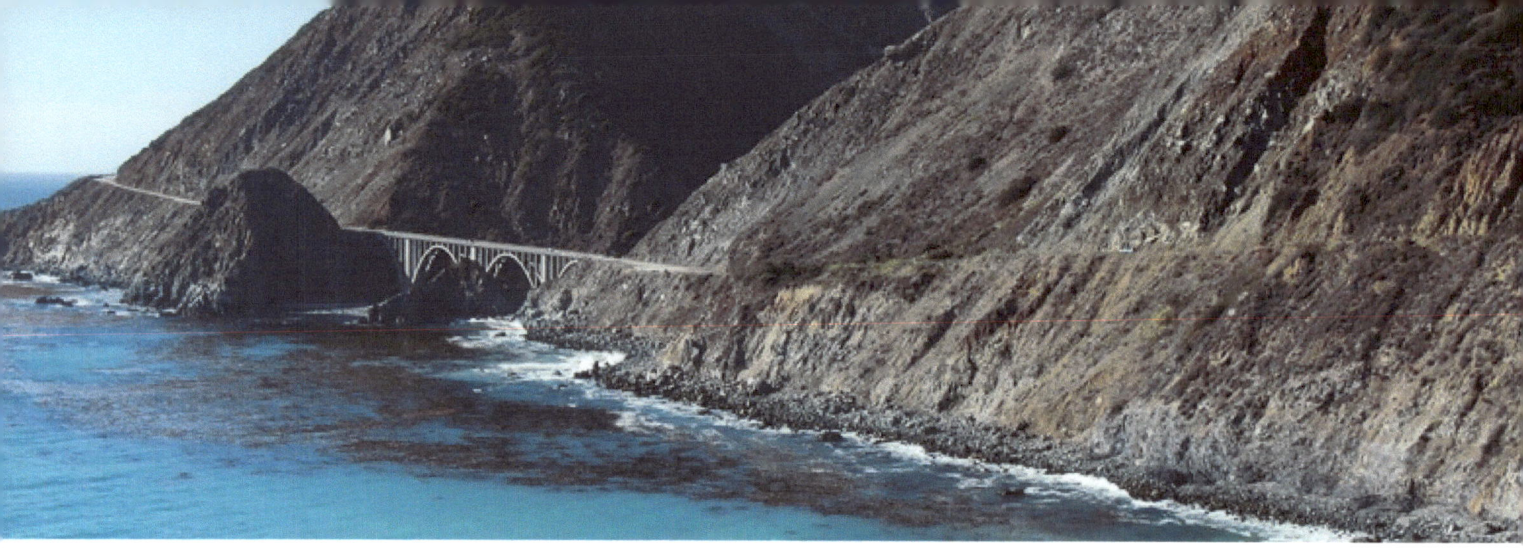

Wheel to the Sea

By Melissa Robison

I really wanted to help. My friend, a fellow veteran, asked me to volunteer for an event where people in wheelchairs are pushed five miles through a canyon trail out to the beach. My buddy, who I do other volunteer work with, leads the event and I wanted to support him. However, I was just so very nervous.

Before the event, I focused on taking my vitamins, sleeping, and yoga stretches. I was excited, but the nervousness lingered. The morning of the Wheel to the Sea event I meditated and set the intention to be in alignment with the universe, help others, and make friends. I buddied up with someone pushing a chair for a disabled female veteran with a super cute service dog named Lucy. The trail was in pretty good shape, though rocky. I had good shoes on, but I have to be careful about where I step because a fall for me is a big deal.

The veteran asked me to take her dog Lucy, and another veteran asked me to take their older pup named Honey Bear, so I now had one pooch zigging and the other dog zagging. They were adorable and soon got in sync, trotting along next to each other. As the participant's wheelchair got stuck in the sand or wedged on rocks, I would lift the front wheels to help keep my team going. On uphill climbs, I assisted in pushing with my free hand and tried to aid other teams as well. About a half mile in, I wondered if I would make it another four and a half miles.

Last year, a group reached out to me to be a wheelchair participant in a similar program. My previous wheelchair bout was just two years ago when I spent nine months in a wheelchair because of another concussion. I later relied on a walker but ended up back in the wheelchair after another surgery, again in the walker, and now I occasionally use a cane but want to throw it out the window most days. Most people don't know that about me because they only see me on my good days. I remembered when I considered entering an event like this a year ago, but the doctors told me not to walk on uneven ground, and because of my other injuries I could only do short and easy hikes.

During the event, my injuries started to put me in severe pain, and I was looking for a spare wheelchair. It always amazes me how many people asked me to help them with lifting or pushing.

Couldn't they tell I am awaiting hip surgery, have a hard time balancing myself, or can barely make it? Of course, they couldn't because I was smiling the whole time. How would anyone know if I did not tell them, yet continue to push on!

The fact that the hike was five miles and not just one mile, really began to mean a lot to me and would make the victory so much greater. It would be an enormous personal success for me while helping others and seeing so many smiles.

Traffic stopped on the Pacific Coast Highway as over one hundred and fifty of us victoriously crossed over to our destination at the beach. The cheers and hugs were just flowing and flowing. I made it - we ALL made it. I pushed my participant over to get lunch and accidentally hit her arm into a table. Bam! All the positive thoughts about my disabilities being at bay came to a sudden halt.

 I have a problem with balance, and I walk into things, so why in the world would I wheel someone around the tables?

Immediately checking on the veteran's arm, and asking if she was okay, I thought about telling her I have a TBI and to excuse my mistake. I opted not to. Apologizing and checking on her well-being was enough, and she genuinely seemed okay.

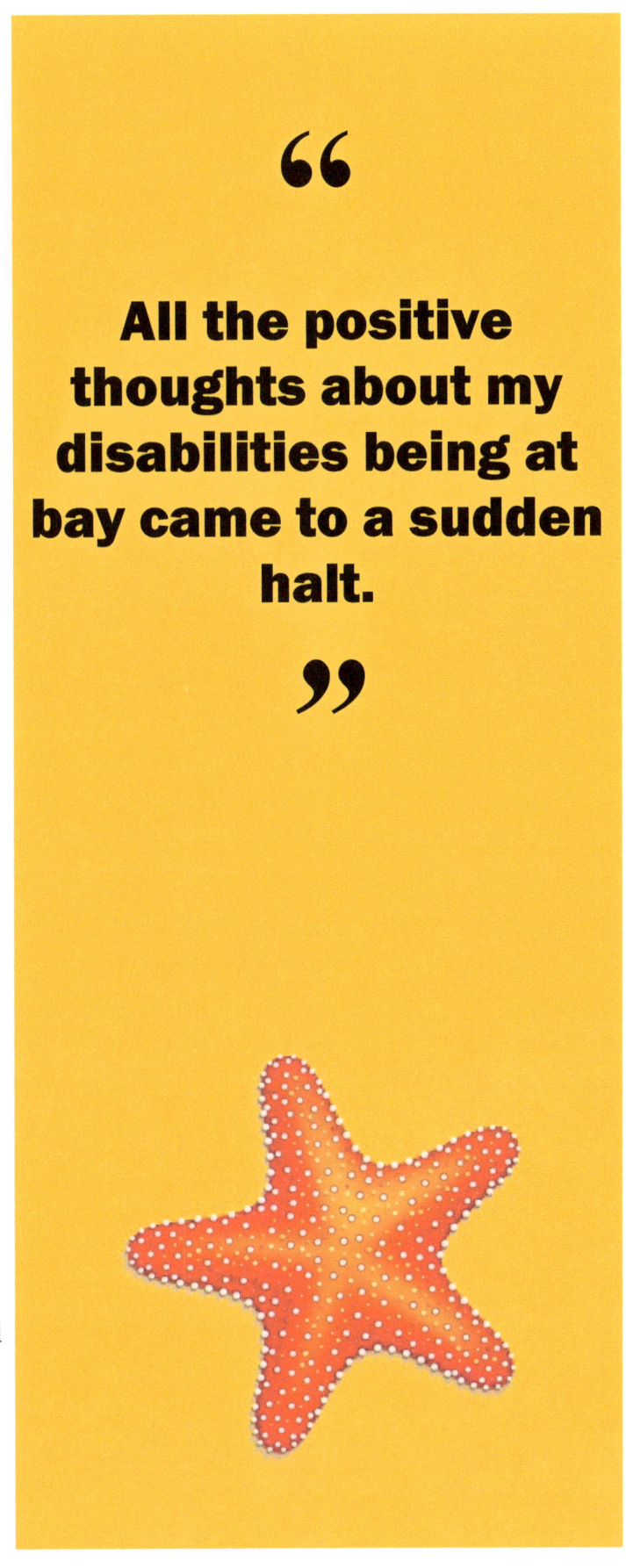

"

All the positive thoughts about my disabilities being at bay came to a sudden halt.

"

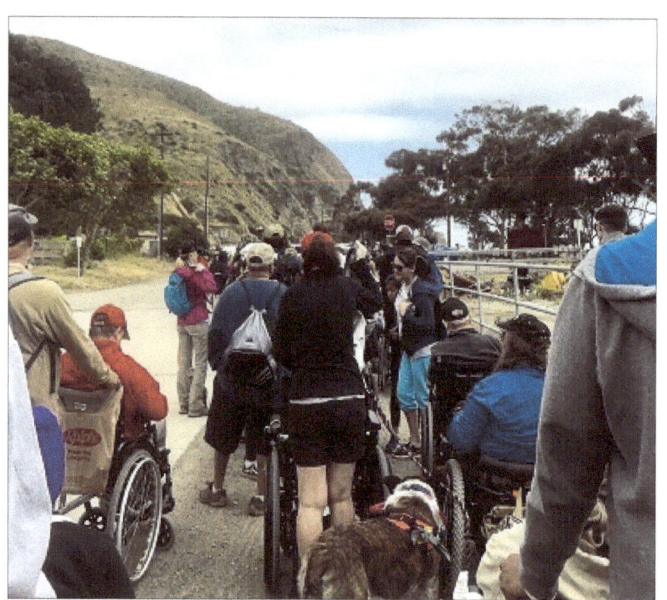

I didn't want to dwell on my symptoms because it serves me better when I focus on all the positives things I do and express gratitude for everything around me. I helped this veteran get her lunch, and she was super happy. With smiles, laughing, and hugs, we all soon went home. Wow, what a day. I felt like I had a new family. I think we all did.

That night, the high of it all was profound. My head kept shaking in disbelief, thinking about the capacity I served in during this event. On the way home, I did pull over to sleep in my car because I was too exhausted to drive. The next morning, I limped into the bath and took some time to reflect. Wow, I've worked so hard on my recovery that I can once again give back and help others. I recognize I've had many ups and downs since my first concussion twenty years ago, and I'm super proud of myself for staying safe yesterday. In the past, before I was aware of my diagnosis, I would not have paid attention to my anxiety, and often pushed myself too hard, causing another injury.

This is a victory I will never forget. I was the person I really wanted so bad to be, during every moment of those down concussion days. I did it. We did as a team. Though completely unaware of what I had been through, my friend's simple request for my help gave me a gift. Each day is a gift, each relationship, and every question posed provides the opportunity to make a choice. I feel like I'm working in step with the world now instead of fighting against it. I was victorious that day, along with everyone else there. We all did the absolute best we could. Amazed, and encouraged, I will do it all again!

Meet Melissa Robison

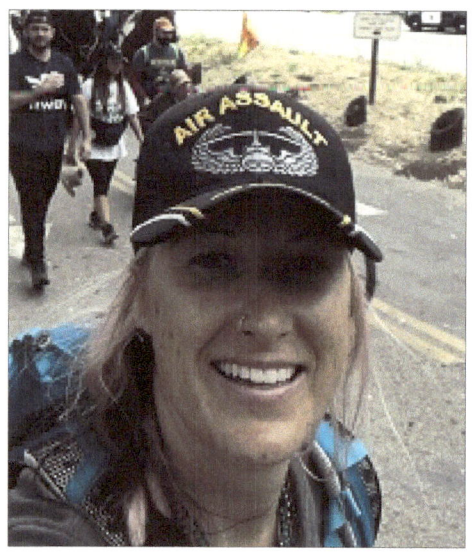

Melissa holds a Bachelor's In Accounting and Master's Degree in Technology Management, she is a recipient of the Massachusetts Women in Public Higher Education Award. A Traumatic Brain Injury and PTSD Survivor, Melissa continues to give compassionately though she has debilitating daily health conditions. Melissa served as a member of a highly respected Spiritual Group in Massachusetts, where she volunteered Medium and Healing services.

Melissa believes she chose this difficult path on this Earth, because she is a server to all of humanity, and will always continue to bring light to those needing it most.

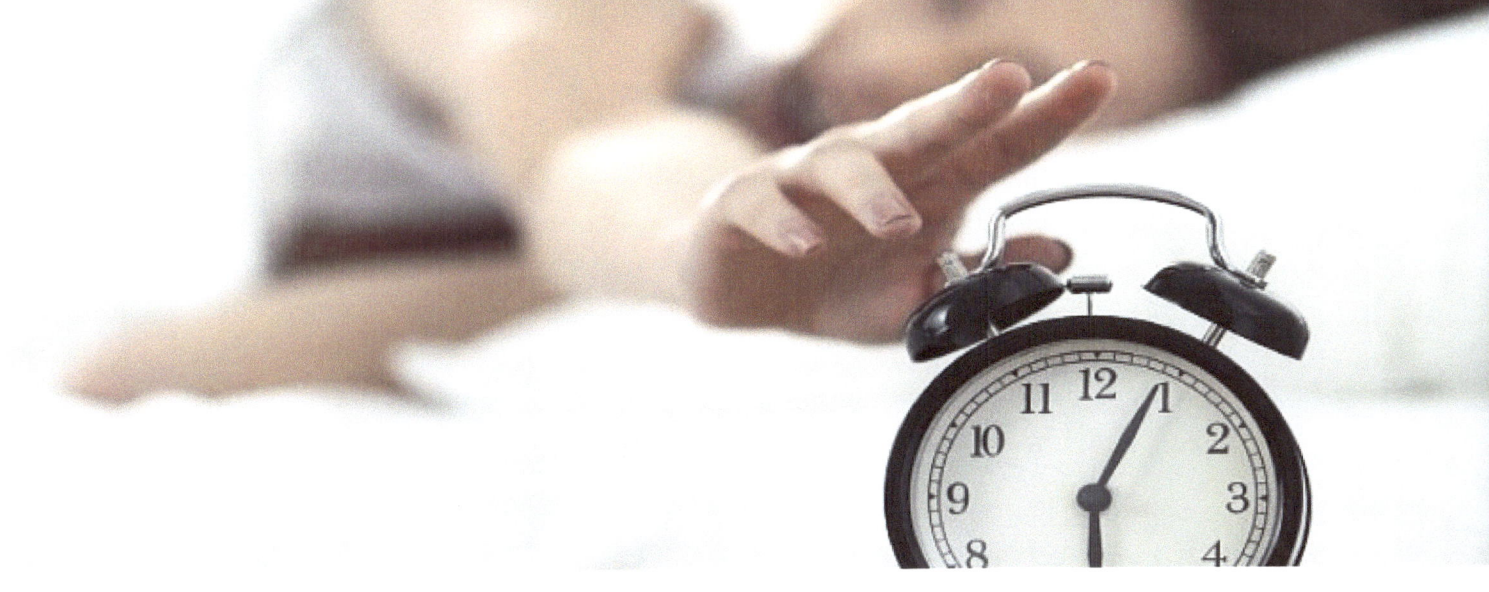

Are You Getting Enough Vitamin Z?

By Barbara Webster

We all know how good it feels to get a good night's sleep or enough "Vitamin Z!" Why is it so hard? Let's face it, when you think about all of the factors that can interfere with sleep, it is a challenge for anyone to get enough sleep, never mind someone who has a brain injury! Typical distractions include things like going off and on daylight savings time, longer days during the summer and a variety of sounds coming through the open windows, changing temperatures, spouses who snore or toss and turn, children or pets in your bed, stress, pain and now blue screens that inhibit melatonin production.

Getting a good night's sleep is especially important for brain injury survivors and the irony is that people with a brain injury often have increased problems getting the quality and quantity of sleep they need! Brain injury often disrupts normal sleep patterns.

I've always been challenged in the sleep department. I'm a "night person" by nature, and I've always needed more than the recommended 7-9 hours of sleep. Then along came some health issues, including my brain injury, and I needed even more sleep. Lately, I've been reading more and more about how important sleep is, specifically for brain function.

For example:

Lack of sleep can interfere with decision-making, creative thinking, contribute to depression, and lead to serious chronic health problems.

Lack of sleep interferes with memory, including the transfer of short-term memory to long-term memory.

Sleep deprivation causes food cravings and an overactive appetite. (Lack of sleep increases the stress hormone cortisol, increasing appetite and cravings for high fat, high carbohydrate foods.

It also boosts levels of ghrelin, the hormone which tells you when you're hungry and decreases the hormone leptin, which signals that satisfied feeling.) Now there is some motivation!

A good night's sleep clears the mind. Research indicates that during sleep, toxic proteins in the brain are washed away, preventing the buildup of plaques that can lead to dementia. Does it get any more important than that?

Without enough sleep, your body and your brain can't restore, repair and rejuvenate.

Ultimately, what is most important about sleep is the quality of it, not the quantity.

According to the experts, there are two essential strategies for getting a good night's sleep:

#1 Maintain regular routines for sleeping and eating: eating meals, going to bed and getting up at the same time each day.

#2 Create a "wind down time" routine before bedtime. Establish relaxing sleep-associated rituals and an electronic curfew one hour before bedtime.

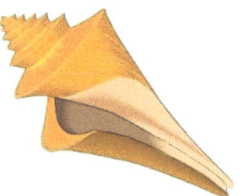

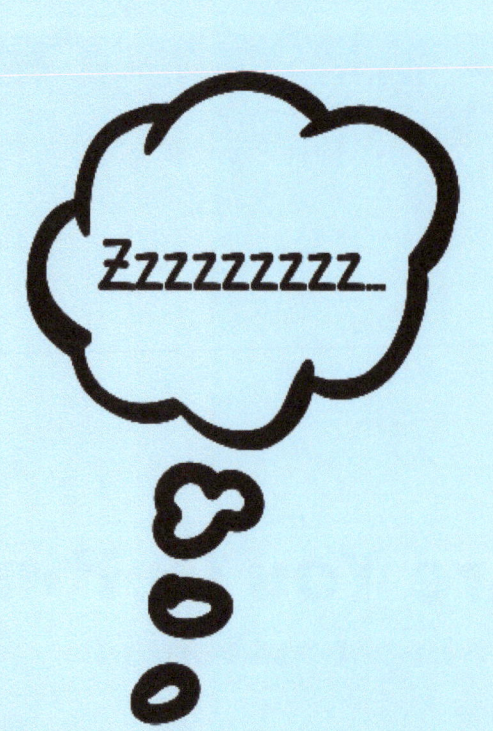

Sleep deprivation causes food cravings and an overactive appetite.

Take a Nap!

Naps are a lost art in our culture, but naps are a good thing. Taking a nap can help to improve mood, alertness, and performance.

Nappers are in good company: Winston Churchill, John F. Kennedy, Ronald Reagan, Napoleon, Albert Einstein, Thomas Edison, and George W. Bush are known to have valued an afternoon nap.

Recommendations include:

▶ Turn off message alerts on phones & computer.

▶ Turn off all electronic devices, notifications, and light sources and charge them in a different room. The blue screens on electronic devices suppress the production of melatonin, a sleep-promoting hormone. (TV is not as bad if watched from a distance.)

▶ Read a physical book. It can help reduce stress by 68%!

▶ Take a hot bath or shower to relax muscles.

▶ Create any routine that works for you, but do it consistently.

Other Practical Strategies:

Most brain injury survivors need a nap or rest break every day. Try not to nap for more than one hour, or after 3:00 pm, to avoid disrupting your sleep cycle.

Take pain medication as prescribed.

Regular exercise, for at least thirty minutes, early in the day: take a walk, walk the dog, gardening, housework, yard work – anything that gets your heart pumping. Avoid exercising late in the day; it sets your body up for activity.

Avoid getting over-tired or pushing yourself on adrenalin. It will be harder to relax, decompress, and fall asleep.

Avoid heavy meals, fatty or spicy foods, and caffeine late in the day, including chocolate (especially dark chocolate)!

Create a relaxing sleep environment – a cool, quiet, dark bedroom. Try playing relaxing music or nature sounds to relax. Try using a fan or white noise machine, or use ear putty to mask background sounds if you are distracted by sounds.

If worrying or trying to remember something keeps you awake, try keeping a small notebook and pencil by your bed where you can jot things down to put your worries on hold for the night.

Meet Barbara Webster

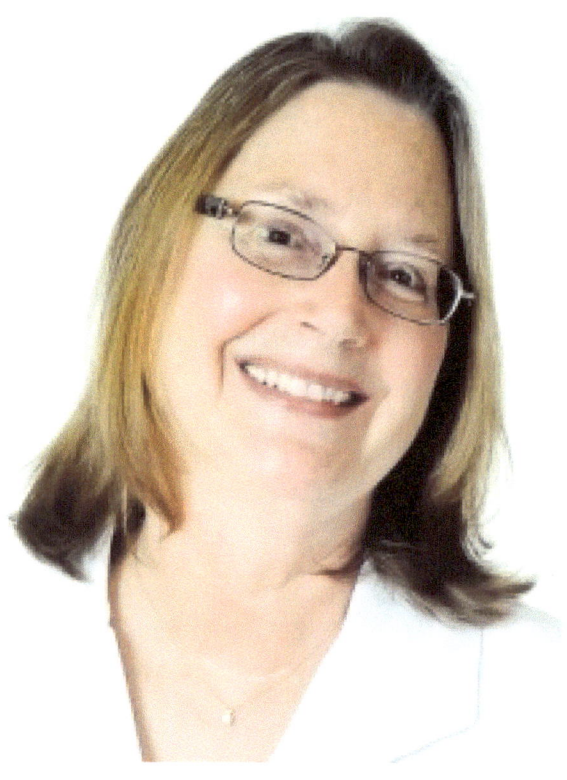

Barbara J. Webster is author of Lost and Found, A Survivors Guide for Reconstructing Life after a Brain Injury, Lash & Assoc. Publishing and a contributor to Chicken Soup for the Traumatic Brain Injury Survivor's Soul.

If all else fails, try counting backward from 300 by three's. It's complicated enough that you can't think of anything else.

So, ask yourself if you are getting enough "Vitamin Z" the next time:

You don't want to get out of bed!
You feel grouchy, irritable, anxious, or emotional
You are particularly sensitive to lights and sounds
You have more trouble than usual focusing, thinking, and making decisions
You make more mistakes than usual
Your balance is off, or you are bumping into things
You are napping more during the day
You are always hungry
You feel depressed

Always check with your doctor to rule out other medical issues that could cause fatigue such as hypothyroidism, anemia, a vitamin deficiency (B12) or medication.

If using these suggestions doesn't help you sleep better, consult your doctor or a sleep specialist.

May you always have plenty of Vitamin Z!

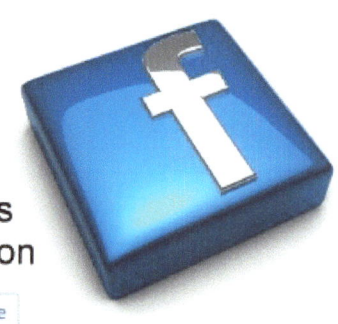

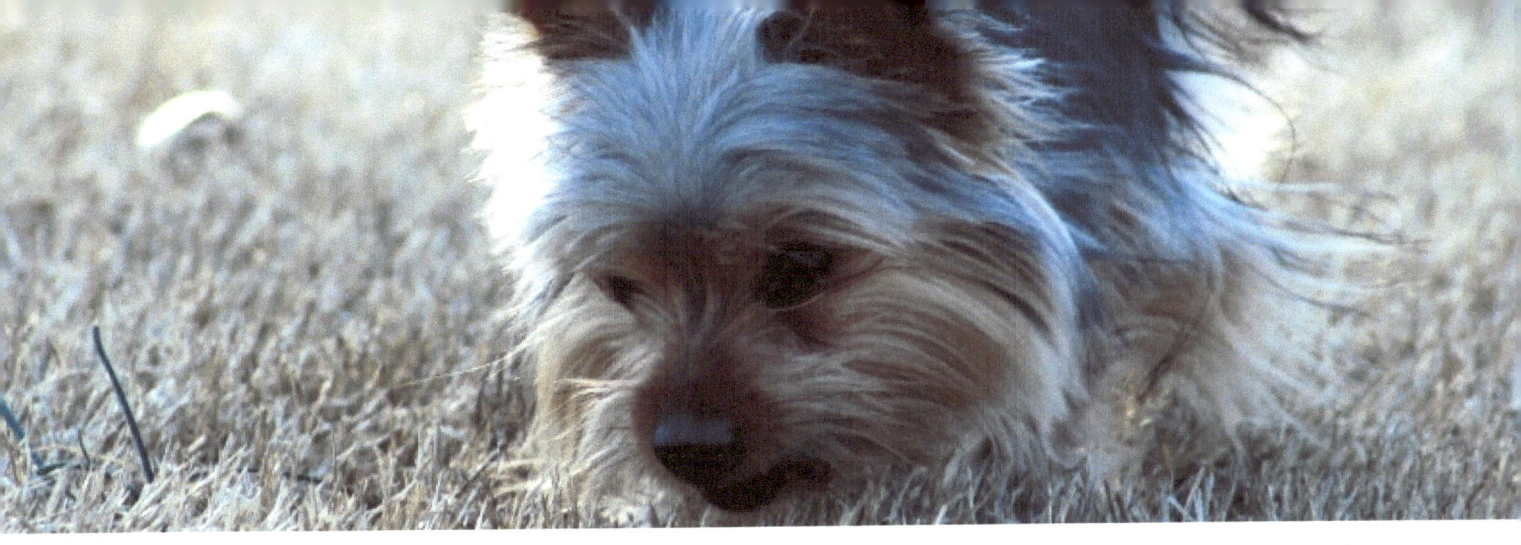

Who Rescued Whom?

By Amy Zellmer

The truth is, I had always been a "cat" woman. I had never owned a dog and had heard how much work they were to take care of, so getting a dog wasn't ever on my radar.
I was recently divorced and feeling a little bit lonely. Even though I had two cats at home, I still felt something was missing in my life. A woman who worked with me would bring her Chihuahua along to the photography studio on Wednesday's—and soon, I was thinking I could handle a little dog.

I reached out to the Carver-Scott Humane Society. A little Yorkie had come into the pound over the weekend. She had been abandoned by the side of the road and was looking a little underweight and shabby. They warned me that she wasn't very friendly, and would bare her teeth at anyone who tried to pick her up, but they were happy to bring her to my home for a meeting.

This lonely, scared little Yorkie showed up at my house and promptly peed in every section of the house. (Was she "marking her territory" because she knew she was staying?) When she finally let me pick her up—she licked my face and looked at me with her big brown eyes. It was pretty much puppy love at first sight.

Pixxie would go with me everywhere dogs were allowed. Friends thought of her more as my child than an actual dog, and even friends who weren't "dog people" would allow her to come to their home, and then say how sweet she was. At the Starbucks drive-thru, her cuteness would command the attention of the entire staff, getting her her very own "pupaccino" (mini cup of whipped cream.) She was also my new road-trip partner – traveling to 36 states and Canada -- and truly my best friend.

Shortly after rescuing her, we moved to a new city where we both quickly settled into our new loft. I was beginning to realize how much of a companion she was for me. Then, on an Arctic-cold February morning, I fell on a patch of ice and landed full force on the back of my skull. Pixxie had been in my arms when I fell. Although she was quite shaken by what had happened, she wasn't hurt. She was sitting

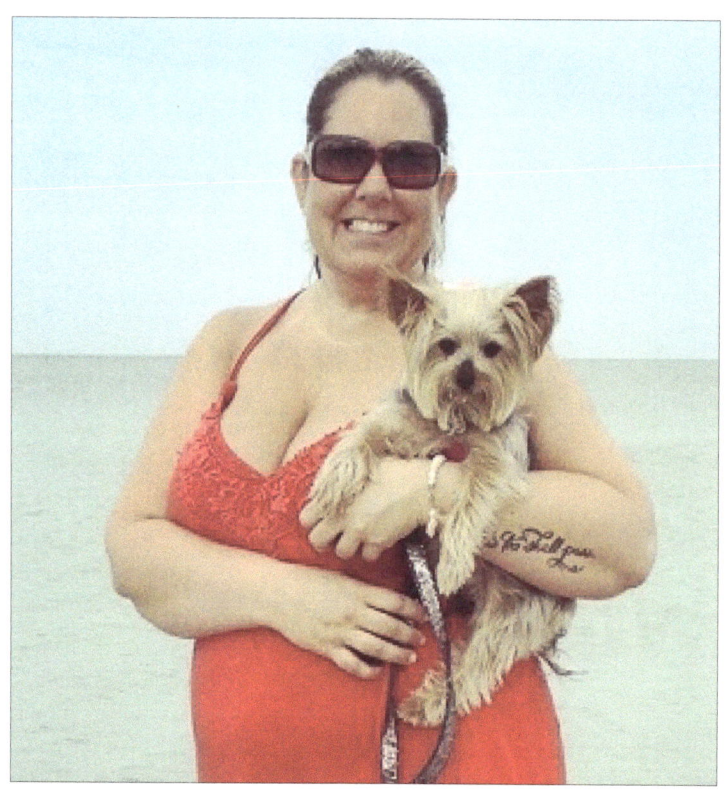

about ten feet from where I lay, looking at me with great "doggy concern," and for a good reason: I had suffered a traumatic brain injury, along with whiplash and a dislocated sternum.

For the first several months, I was completely dazed and confused and would sleep for 12–14 hours at night. At first, I was worried that Pixxie would have a potty accident being in the bedroom during my long night's sleep, but she didn't. She knew I wasn't okay and would give me extra snuggles and puppy kisses, and let me sleep in as late as I needed. Pixxie could sense when I was in a lot of pain or was feeling depressed, and she would always come to my rescue, giving me reassuring licks after crawling up onto my lap. Even in my darkest days, she was by my side with those big ol' puppy eyes, letting me know that she was there for me—even if I couldn't remember whether or not I had fed her dinner yet. She was my motivation to get up in the morning, and having a routine to take her out for her morning walk was a godsend.

I firmly believe having Pixxie kept me going when things got hard. If I was frustrated or confused, sad or lonely, I would hear the sweet sounds of the little Yorkie I rescued only a year earlier. It's tough to be sad when a dog is licking your face!

While I rescued Pixxie from a life of abandonment and mistreatment, I believe she came into my life at just the right time to rescue me from an unexpected accident and period of darkness.
It's the proverbial cliché – who rescued whom?

Meet Amy Zellmer

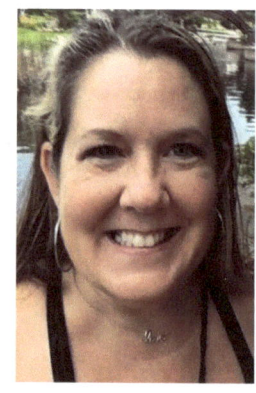

In February 2014 Amy Zellmer slipped on a patch of ice and fell, forcibly landing on the back of her skull. Amy had suffered a Traumatic Brain Injury (TBI) and was about to started a journey unlike anything she had ever experienced. Today, Amy is a writer, photographer, coach, and TBI survivor. Located in Saint Paul, MN she is a regular contributor for the Huffington Post. She enjoys traveling the country with her Yorkie named Pixxie. She loves chocolate, Miss Me jeans, Starbucks, and everything glittery and sparkly.

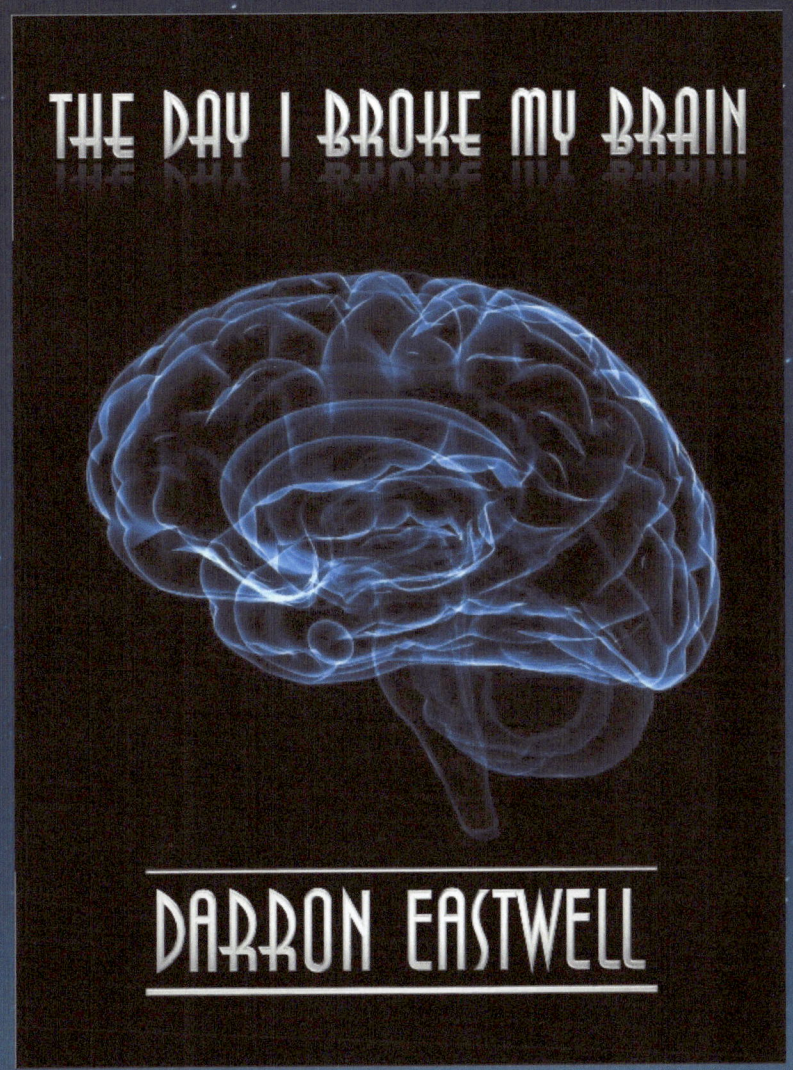

NOW AVAILABLE

THE DAY I BROKE MY BRAIN

DARRON EASTWELL

AN INSPIRATIONAL NEW BOOK BY SURVIVOR

DARRON EASTWELL

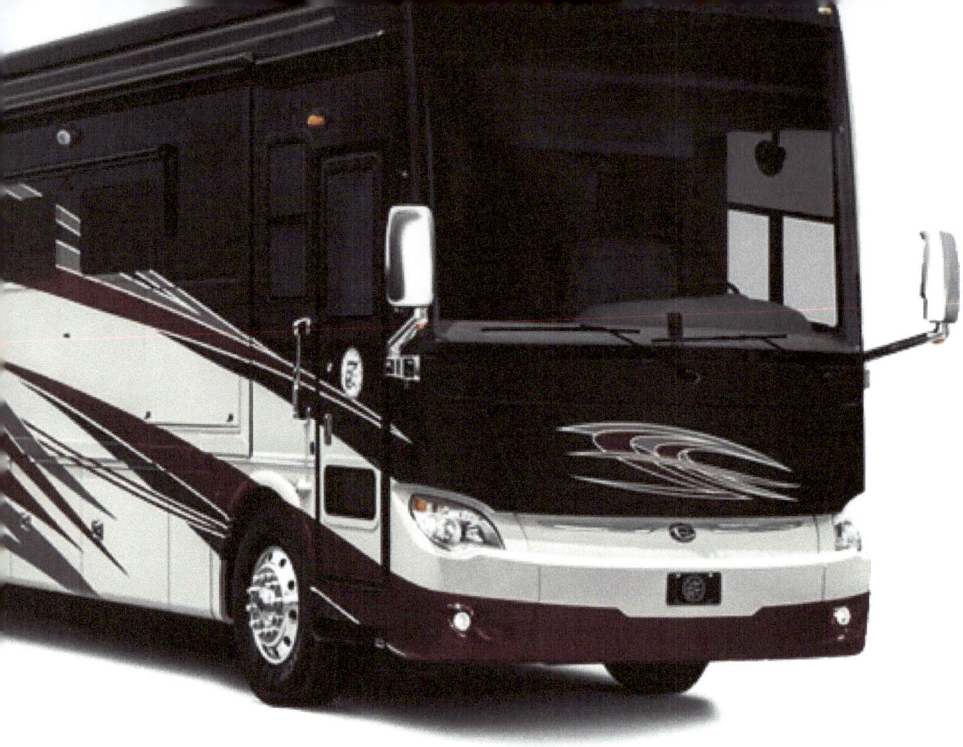

Because I Can!

By Rosalie Johnson

When I go to Florida in my motorhome, it's a fresh start. Each day is planned and planned again, well in advance, using the strategies I learned while recovering from a Traumatic Brain Injury.

On the road, I can only move forward. I can still remember my other life: work, volunteer, play, maintain a home and still have plenty of time to spend with my husband Randy, family, and friends.

Like most survivors, I remember when that world crashed – December 8, 2001. In my new reality, I feel as if I am a child's toy top spinning so fast that the centrifugal force is randomly spewing away my thoughts and plans to be productive. Some days the top slows down, and on others, it rotates so quickly that it is all I can do just to hang on and ride.

Travel gives me back control. With my itinerary plan and the larders stocked, Randy tries to start the trip with me. We head south in the late winter. Each day we drive 250-300 miles easing into a routine, and trying to miss any snowstorm in the forecast. Arriving at an RV campground, we level the motorhome, extend the slides, and connect the water and sewer.

Next, I walk the "Road Warrior" – my old Yorkie, Lilly. Then there is dinner to prepare, clean up, and finally sleep. The next morning the routine is reversed. Any items we used must be stowed, as they become projectiles while traveling. At some airport along the route, I usually have to drop Randy off to fly home so he can return to work. You should see some of the looks we get when driving our motorhome through the departure area of an airport! Being a pilot, he will be able to meet me at future destinations down the road.

I spend a week here or two weeks there, eventually making it all the way to Key West. Every day is planned, such as stopping for gas or groceries along the way, because once the RV is parked and set up, I can't just drive to any store. I get around on my bicycle for planned adventures.

I am very fortunate to have family and friends join me along the way. I love the company for exploring new areas but there is one stipulation: they have to be ready to bicycle or walk everywhere. Just ask my friend, Anne, about her "Vacation Boot Camp!" I have baskets and coolers to attach to our bicycles, along with a cart to carry groceries, laundry, or beach chairs.

When traveling alone, I am rarely lonely. Walking Lilly, I meet many other dogs. Each evening finds most campers at the waterfront to marvel at the beauty of the sunset. More bonds form. The people I encounter are from all over the world, and all share the same bond: "Wanderlust." In meeting so many interesting folks, the number of Traumatic Brain Injury and Stroke survivors is astounding.

With one particular couple, the wife suffered a stroke some years ago. Each evening her husband bundles her up and helps her into their golf cart, then drives to the waterfront to watch the sunset. Due to the severity of her aphasia, she is only able to speak three words. She will take each person's hand, place it on her heart, look deeply into their eyes and say "I love you, I LOVE YOU!" Is there any better way to share a sunset?

Along the way, I'm invited to join other RV'ers for potluck dinners, Yoga, airplane rides, museum tours, and much, much more. The people I have the pleasure to meet share so much of their lives with me. They are like little gifts. Each day I learn something new: the name of a flower or tree, or the mating habits of dolphins or alligators.

When learning that I am a Traumatic Brain Injury survivor, many other travelers will ask me how I can drive the RV and do all of the set up mostly alone. I respond, "Because I can!"

Meet Rosalie Johnson

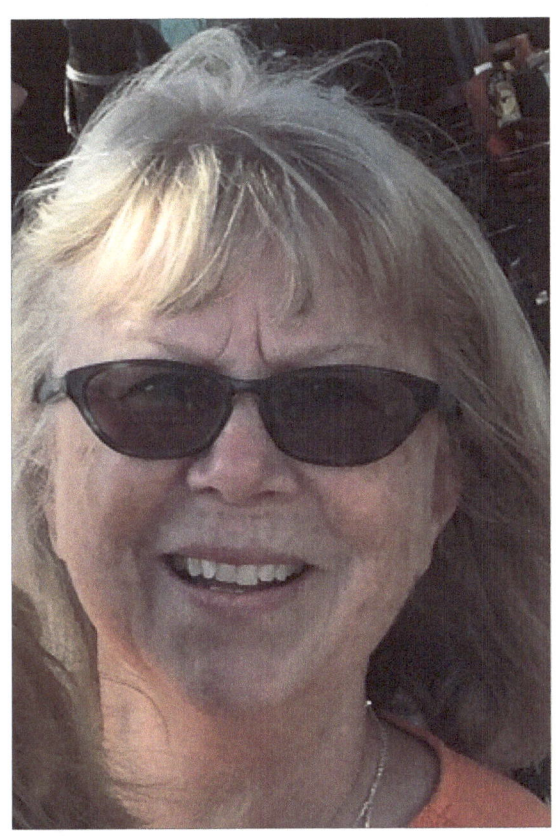

Before her Traumatic Brain Injury, Rosalie Johnson was a Registered Nurse and loved volunteering for various non-profit organizations. She was able to travel, and live and work throughout the country with her husband, Randy and their ever changing family of dogs.

These days Rosalie can be found running the Seacoast Brain Injury Support Group and volunteering at Krempels Center in Portsmouth, New Hampshire. She is a seven-year Board Member for the Brain Injury Association of New Hampshire, author of "Meet the Artist" article printed quarterly in HEADWAY Newsletter published by BIANH. She is also a liaison with the BIANH and Camp Allen in Bedford, NH, organizing a three night and four day camping adventures for adult TBI survivors.

And if you can't find her, she is probably on the road traveling in her motorhome!

Check Out The Newly Expanded

The TBI HOPE Book Directory

A comprehensive list of TBI books by survivors and those who love them!

Featuring "The Best of the Best!"

www.TBIBooks.org

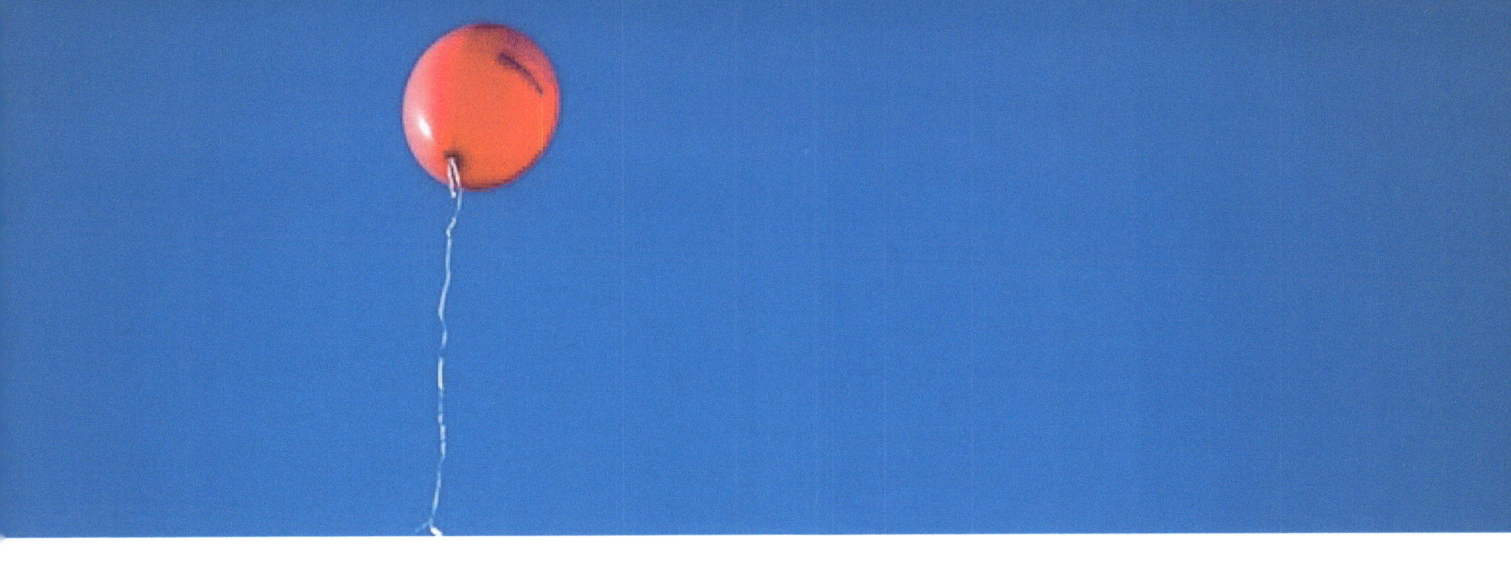

Letting go is Hard

By Jen Dodge

I've never considered myself a high maintenance person or a materialistic person. I'm happier sitting around a campfire than I am with a fancy dinner out. I'm more comfortable wearing jeans than I am in high heels. I'd rather you bring me a coffee how I drink it, versus a dozen roses. I think you get where I'm heading with this.

Since the ripe old' age of...however old you are when you start thinking about life as an adult...there have only been a few things I wanted. I wanted to be a special education teacher (I've known this was my passion since the age of eight). I wanted a husband to laugh and grow old with. I wanted a couple of children (here is a separate confession for you: since I was a teen, I've thought of boy's and girl's names that I would like for my unborn children). I wanted the dog that's outside playing in the yard with the kids.

I never cared about the kind of house we would live in (yes that cabin by the lake would be beautiful, but it could also be a double-wide trailer for all I cared. What mattered was the happiness inside the house.) I never cared about the kind of car we drove (if it got us from point A to point B and the children didn't fall through holes in the floorboards, the rest didn't matter to me.)

As I got older, those dreams morphed slightly, showing me the specifics of what I wanted and what I did not want. For instance, my ideal husband became someone athletic so we could hike, bike, and ski together.

My point is that I've never wanted much.

Since August 19, 2014, I have slowly let some dreams go. These simple ideas of mine no longer aligned with my rattled head. Kids? How in the world do you have children when you sleep so much, and noise overwhelms you? I think people have misunderstood me when I've said this in the past. It's not just an infant that seems out of the question; it's a small human being who would depend on me. Eight-years-old or eight-months-old, me sleeping ten to twelve hours a night would be out of the question. Having a "bad rattled head day" and staying on the couch would no longer be an option. The stress, the noise, the stimulation of a child are all things I try to limit or avoid on a daily basis because they are triggers for me. So tell me how that could work?

Perhaps being a wife is still an option (I'll leave out the fact that the dating pool in this area is shallow and filled with deformed fish!) but it's hard to become a wife when dating with a head injury presents its own challenges. It's a rare gift to find someone tolerant of your "new" life, or someone who understands your need for sleep and quiet. Someone who doesn't hold a grudge for canceling last minute and someone who's okay with lots of nights "in" because restaurants can be a nightmare. How do you talk about your head injury and be open and honest about it, without scaring the guy away? It's hard to be comfortable enough to let your guard down and show them what a mess you are because pretending that you're okay 24/7 is exhausting. Call me crazy, but I no longer see this happening for me either.

From Day One, I struggled to work as a special education teacher with a head injury. I did my job, but it cost me. I'll even go so far as to say I was still a good teacher, but I wasn't as good as I used to be. I gave everything at work, but there was nothing left afterward. I'd crawl in the door after a day of teaching, eat a bowl of cereal, and go to bed. My brain was done! It wasn't a life, but I so badly wanted to continue teaching.

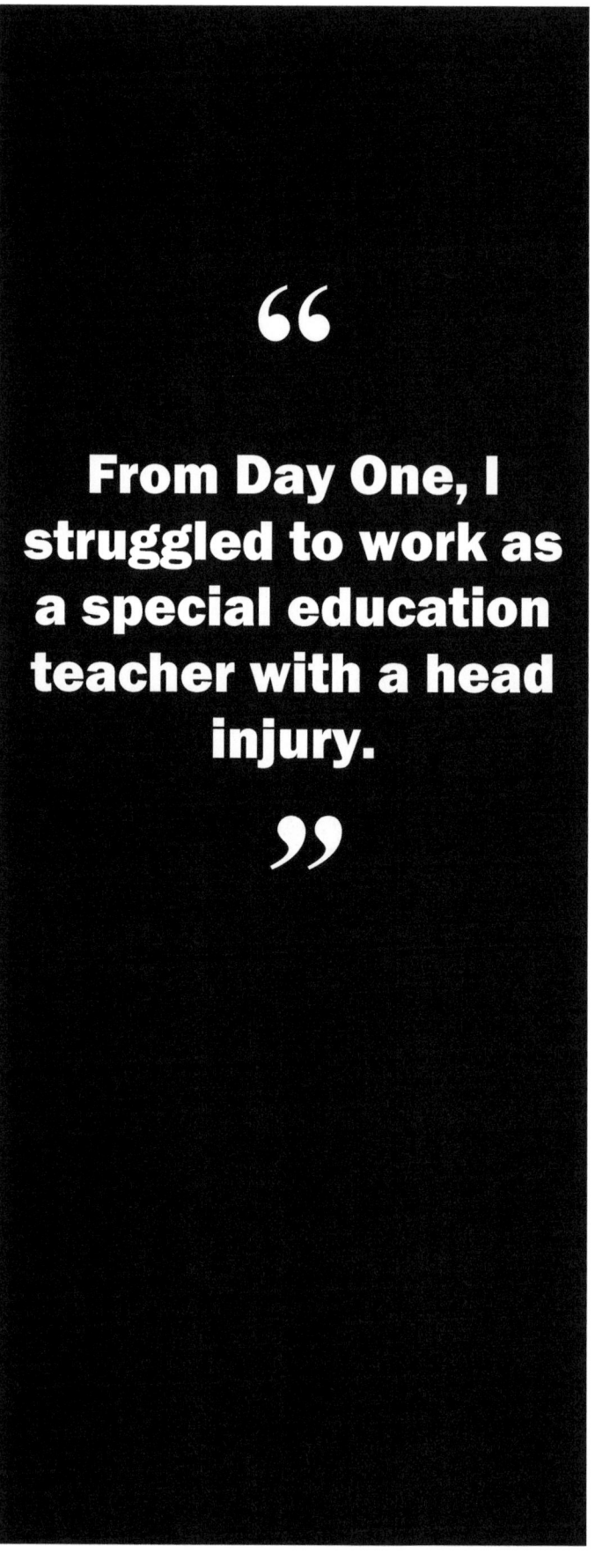

" From Day One, I struggled to work as a special education teacher with a head injury. "

Teaching is natural for me; it comes easily to me. I've spent my life preparing for it. I did not want a head injury to prevent me from doing what I loved. But it did. In the end, the head injury cost me my job. I had pushed so hard for two years post-accident, that when I finally stopped and allowed myself a break, I crashed. I crashed hard! I knew continuing to teach after the accident was taking a toll on me, I just didn't realize how much of a toll it was, until I was forced to stop.

I still hope to return to it. But even now, with ten months of not teaching and giving my head a break, as soon as the going gets tough, and as soon as my stress level rises or my day is too busy, or even if I'm just too tired, my brain shuts down. Nothing has changed in ten months.

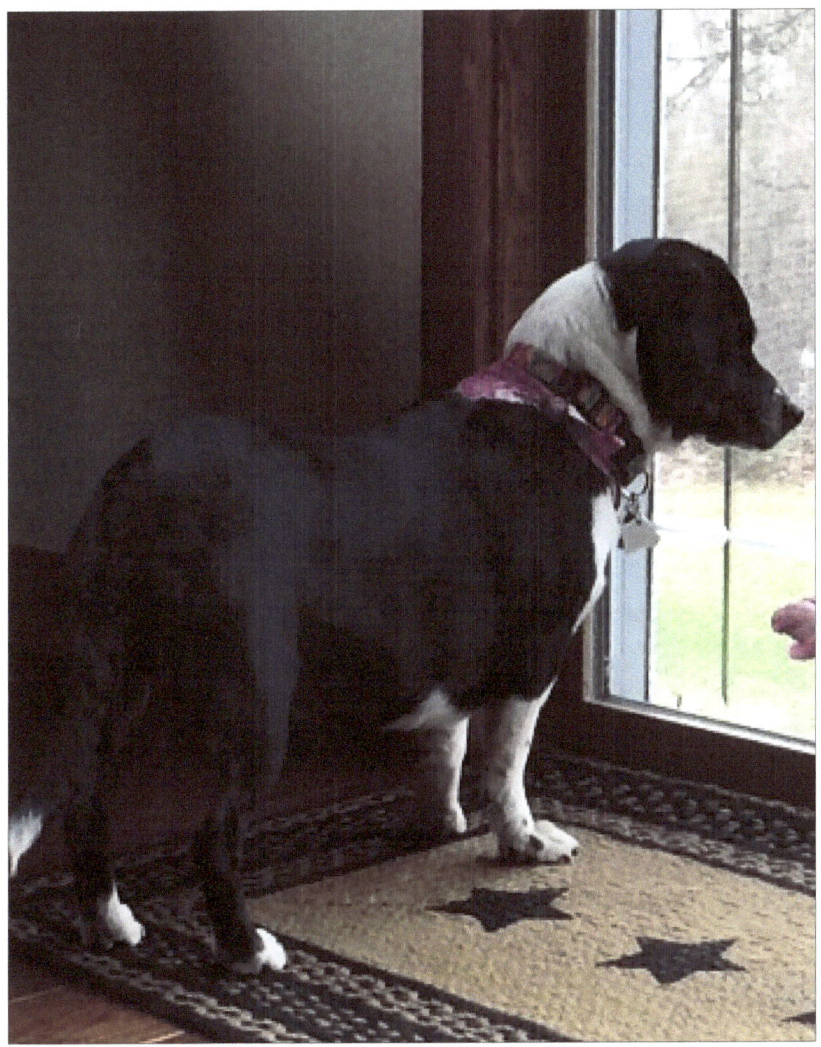

The last thing I always dreamed of having, that is now off my list, is a dog. Theoretically, this should have been the easiest thing on the list, but it was still too hard for my broken brain. Everyone had something to say about it (in this day and age, everyone has something to say to everything, without always knowing the full story) and many sold me short in the long-run. "Dogs are easy," and "just find one that doesn't have medical needs," etc.

The overall problem I found by fostering a dog, and I learned this lesson quickly, was that she consumed my thoughts: does she need to go out? Is it time for her to eat? She needs her insulin shot in twenty minutes. Check her for ticks!

Even when I was exhausted and needed to rest, she wanted love, attention, a walk, etc. None of that sounds like much, but it all takes mental energy (which is something extra taxing for a rattled brain). I was feeling sorry because I couldn't keep my foster pup and I felt pretty weak that even having a tiny, easy-go-lucky dog was too much for me when I spoke to one of my favorite people about how I was wearing down, and he said "Of course you are! Dogs are a lot of work. They take up a lot of mental energy, and this would be even worse on you." I can always count on him to understand. I'm allergic to cats, so although they are pretty low-maintenance, they are out of the question. Perhaps I'm destined only to own a goldfish.

Every time I've had to cross off something on my "wish list of life," and every time I've had to let go of a dream, it hurts. It's like a death. I need time to mourn it. Everything just comes crashing back down on me: the anger, the hurt, and frustration about that awful August day. It's a lot to deal with. It's a lot to process and accept. Some days are better than others.

I've never once written a Confession looking for sympathy. I write them as a form of coping for myself and informing those around me. It's impossible to put into words what it's like living with a brain injury, and it's equally impossible to put into words how it has affected me (and how it continues to affect me).

So, if you've made it this far in this Confession, do me a favor. Hug your spouse and be thankful for their love every single day. Tell your kids how thankful you are for them and never forget it. Get on the floor and rub your dog's stomach until your arms ache. And go to work on Monday, thankful to be doing a job you love.

Meet Jen Dodge

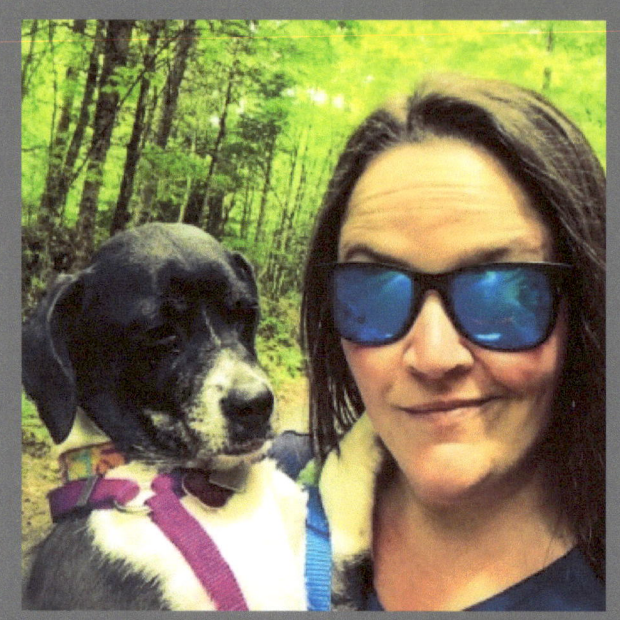

Jen is a 34 year old resident of northern New Hampshire. On August 19, 2014, she was hit by an SUV while riding her bicycle on a group ride. Since the accident she has written several articles titled "Confessions of a Concussed Cyclist" to help inform others and as a form of therapy for herself. She is a certified Special Education teacher, and an avid cyclist. Jen uses her own story to encourage people to become informed about the invisible disability of a brain injury and to be kind to cyclists and Share the Road!

When you come out of the storm you won't be the same person that walked in. That's what the storm is all about.

~Haruki Murakami

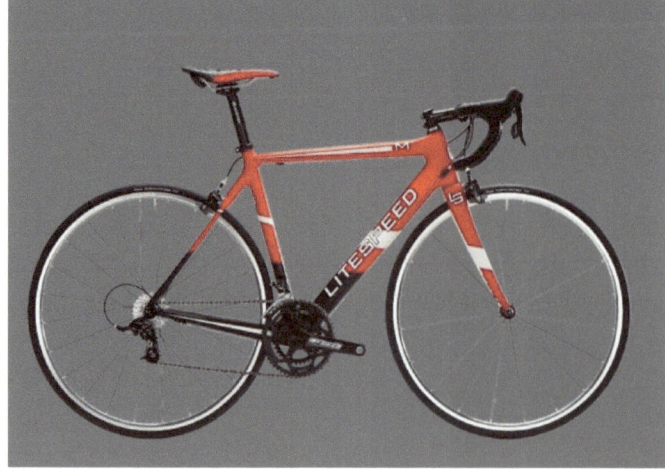

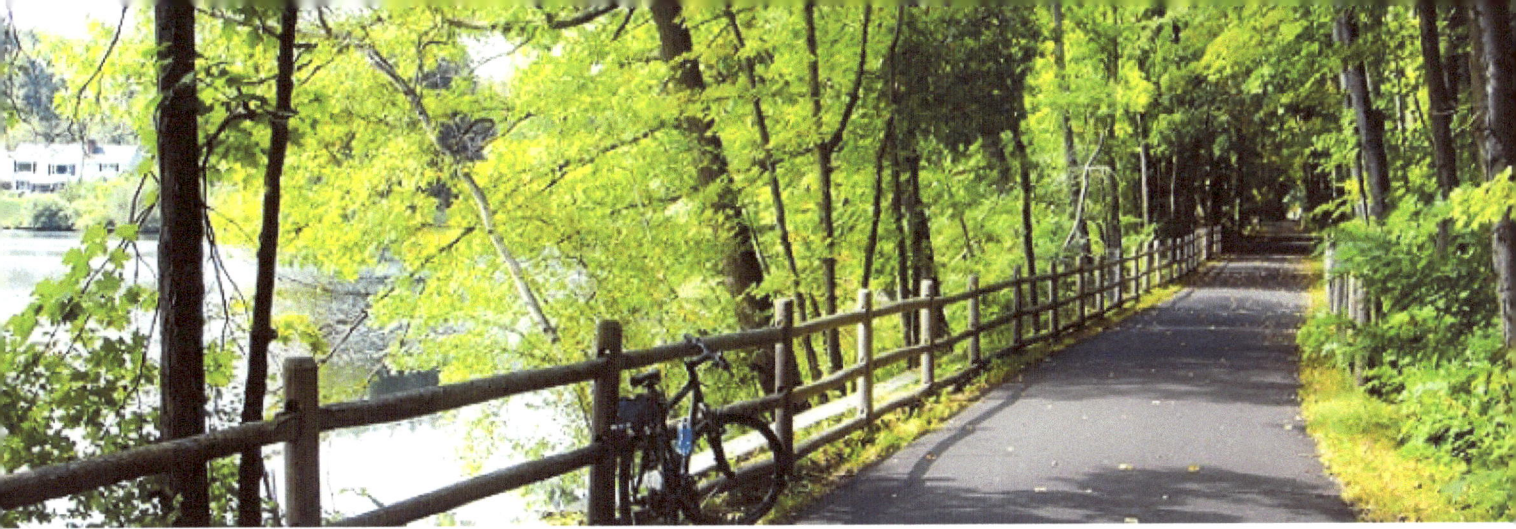

Setting Goals & Staying Active

By Derek O'Brien

My name is Derek O'Brien. July 23, 2005, was the day that my life changed forever. When I was a 4th-year architecture student, I was celebrating college break in New Jersey. I dove headfirst into a sandbar and became a quadriplegic after breaking my neck at c6-c7.

Luckily, a nurse who witnessed my accident insisted that I be raced to a trauma unit, where I was put into a medically-induced coma. When I remained unresponsive, I was airlifted to Massachusetts General Hospital. The treatment I received there finally woke me up from my coma. After I woke up, I had to relearn everything. I engaged in years of rehabilitation from inpatient to outpatient therapy and even traveled to China for stem cell replacement. Those years of treatment and therapy led me to where I am today – living independently.

The next direction in my life was to return to college to pursue my new-found passion for new media and photography. I enrolled in the University of Maine and graduated with a BA. While I was in college, I started a personal project taking a photograph a day. The project led me to complete four consecutive years of a photo-a-day, using a different device each year.

> **"After I woke up, I had to relearn everything."**

In the summer of 2012, I was a camp counselor at Empower SCI – a camp for adults with spinal cord injury. I did that for three summers. There is no better feeling than showing newly injured people that though they are injured, life is not over.

I am currently living in Portland, Maine in my own apartment. I work part-time as a video editor for a local television station. I am also on the board of directors for Alpha One, an independent living center of Southern Maine.

The most important lesson I have learned from my brain injury is the importance of setting goals and staying active. Life is short. Do not let anybody tell you can't do something. You can overcome anything.

Meet Derek O'Brien

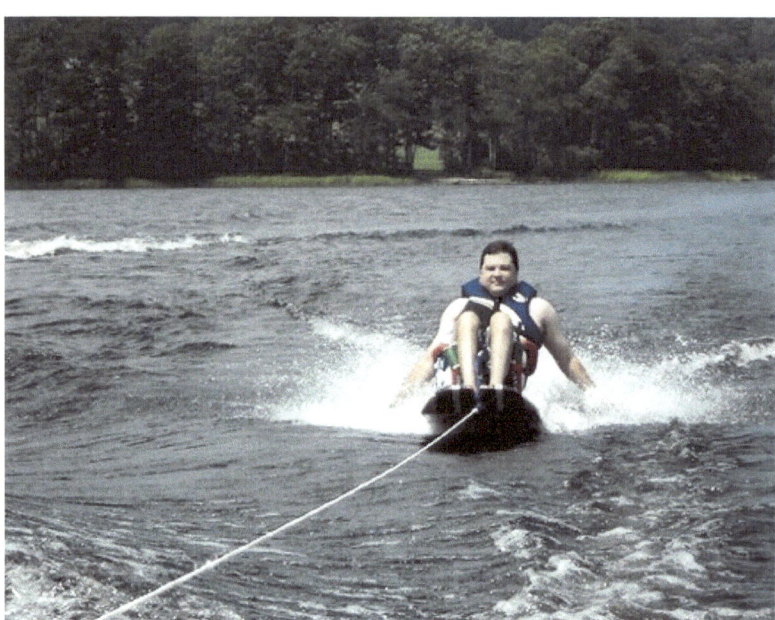

Derek O'Brien is from Rockport, Maine. He is a quadriplegic. Derek broke his neck on July 23, 2005 at c6-c7 after a diving accident. Derek studied photography during high school and majored in architecture at Catholic University of America. After his hospital stay, he resumed photography and completed a four year photo-a-day project. Derek went on to attend college at UMaine studying New Media and graduated in 2013. He was also a camp counselor at Empower a camp for adults with spinal cord injury. Derek currently lives in Portland Maine working for CTN as video editor.

Living With Hope

By Patrick Brigham

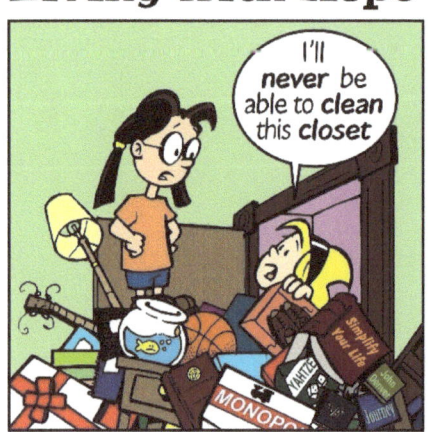
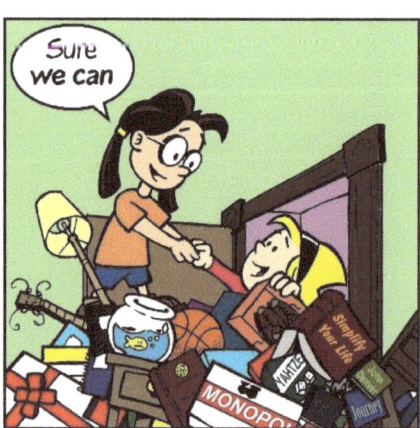
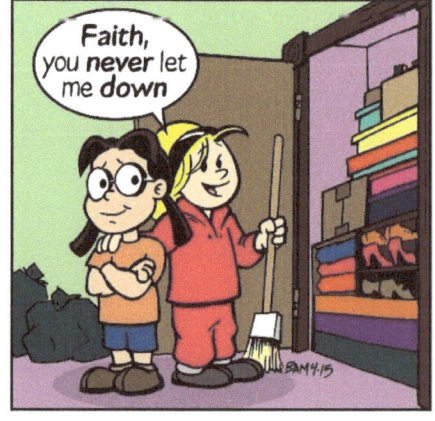

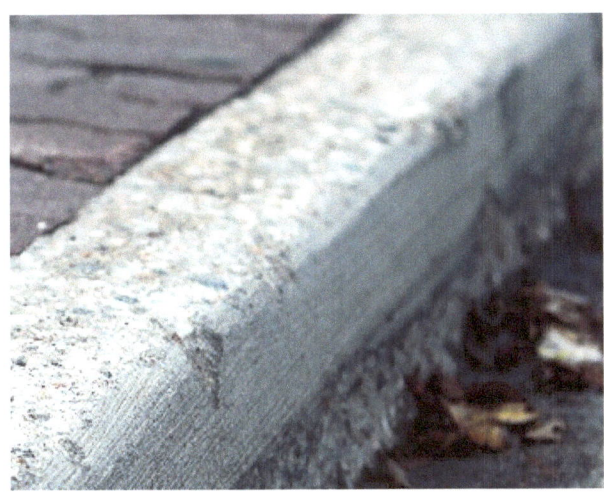

I Stumbled but Did Not Fall

By Donna O'Donnell Figurski

Recently, as I got out of my car, I stumbled on the curb. Somehow in the darkness, I did not see it. Though the event took less than a second, one thought ran through my head. It was not, "Oh, no! I am going to break a bone or scrape my knee." It was not, "What a klutz! I'll ruin my clothes." And it was not about how embarrassed I would be. All of those possibilities probably would have been my first thoughts before brain injury entered my life in 2005 when my husband had a traumatic brain injury.

Now my mind is only a thought away from brain injury. So, as I tripped and stumbled, but did not fall, I thought, "Please don't let me hit my head." I didn't care how silly I looked or about my clothes being ripped or about getting any broken bones (they would heal). I was concerned about getting a brain injury. I worried about how a brain injury could change my life forever. I worried that if I were hurt, I could not sufficiently care for my husband, who needs my daily attention. Yes, those thoughts raced through my head in that fleeting second. It only takes a second for a brain injury to occur. Most brain injuries occur because of an accident. Though we may be aware of the possibility of accidents, we cannot avoid all of them. Fortunately, my accident was avoided – just barely. I can only hope that my potential accidents will be few and far apart in the future. I hope yours will be too.

Meet Donna O'Donnell Figurski

Donna O'Donnell Figurski, whose life revolves around traumatic brain injury (TBI), is a wife, mother, granny, teacher, playwright, actor, director, picture-book reviewer, radio host, speaker, photographer, and writer.

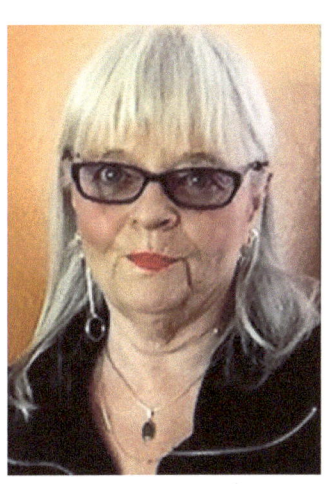

As a brain injury advocate, Donna has published articles in many brain-injury-related magazines on the web; has written chapters included in two books; writes a blog called "Surviving Traumatic Brain Injury"; is host of her international radio show, "Another Fork in the Road," online on the Brain Injury Radio Network, and is a speaker concerned with survivors of brain injury and their caregivers.

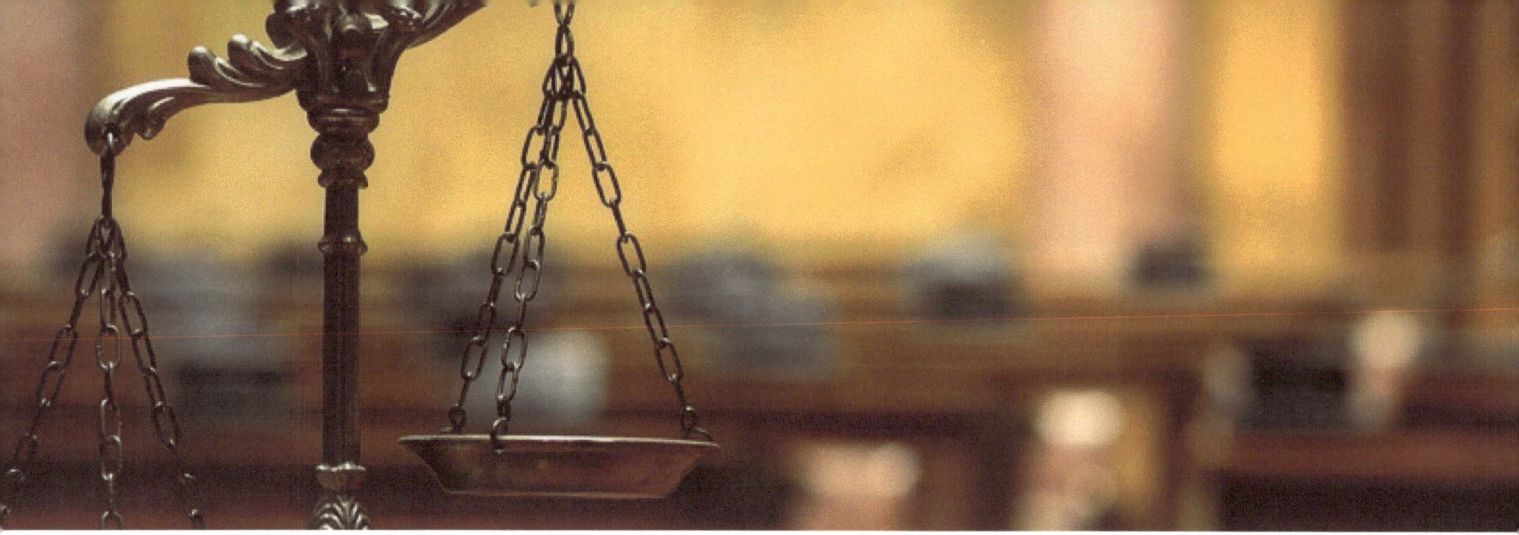

The Importance of Hope

By Jim Martin

Before December 2010, I enjoyed a successful professional career as an active trial lawyer, primarily representing physicians in medical malpractice litigation, and municipalities in many forms of civil litigation including employment matters, civil rights, alleged police misconduct and others. It was a rewarding and, in retrospect, an all-consuming life adventure.

In December 2010, although I have no memory whatsoever, I experienced a traumatic brain injury in which I was apparently unconscious for 22-24 hours. Spending six weeks in various hospitals, including RIO at Good Samaritan Hospital, I then spent three months in a foster care home specializing in brain injury patients. Then, thinking I was healed and would be returning to my trial practice, I was confronted with multiple medical opinions which suggested, given my permanent memory impairment, it would not be wise to place a client's interest at risk. I was advised not to return to work. Subsequently, the Social Security Administration determined that I was disabled for purposes of receiving disability benefits. Then, the painfully slow process of attempting to return to normalcy followed.

> **"My physical limitations seemed to exacerbate my memory and concentration impairments."**

By this time in early 2013, my children were young adults and moved on to other cities and countries to pursue their dreams. My wife at the time had relocated her retail business from Portland to Bend, and our social network was evaporating. Also, I underwent nine surgeries since April 2013, as a result of the accident which caused my brain injury.

My physical limitations seemed to exacerbate my memory and concentration impairments. With encouragement, I was able to volunteer at a local hospital, the Alzheimer's Association, and as a Mentor in the Oregon State Bar Mentor/Mentee program. The latter permitted me to share my previous experiences and maintain contacts with several other lawyers, judges, and friends in the legal community.

Recently, I've become more active in a support group for brain injury survivors, which has permitted me to address the potential effects and complications of returning to my legal practice. For example, with the possible risk of developing earlier than usual onset of dementia, regardless of cause, I needed to be very aware of the potential effects on clients and partners, colleagues and staff.

Nonetheless, despite being somewhat helpful to several individuals, I also recognized that apathy was prevalent in perspective of my external world. Stated differently, I perceived that I lost the identity of who I was and the significance my efforts were making for others.

Throughout the past five years post-accident, and even more recently, I've come to realize the importance of sustaining hope, which has been described for me as follows: Hope is born while facing the unknown and discovering that one is not alone.

Hope is not a concept easily defined. I've managed to achieve a sense of contentment, which, for me, is an awareness of sufficiency; a feeling that we have enough and we are enough. It means appreciating the simple gifts of life - friendship, books, a good laugh, a moment of beauty, a cold drink on a hot day. Being content, we are free from the pull of greed and longing. We trust that life provides what we need when we need it.

Contentment allows us to experience satisfaction with what is. We are fully present in this moment. Being content does not obstruct our dreams or thwart our purpose. It is a place to stand and view the future with a peaceful heart and gratitude for all that is and all that is to come.

> " Contentment allows us to experience satisfaction with what is. "

Surely, my life is at least 180 degrees from where it was before December 2010.

Personally, professionally, and physically, everything is different. Recognizing this period of time as one of transition rather than change has allowed me to maintain a sense of balance and realize that there may yet be productive and beneficial opportunities which lie ahead and may afford me an opportunity to be effective in some other manner, the nature and extent of which is not yet evident. Balance in this context is the awareness that "falling short" implies two related realities: First, we are trying, and second, we need to try again.

There is no failure here because spirituality involves a continual falling down and getting back up again. The great need is for balance - when we are down, we need to get back up, and when we are up, we need to remember that we have been, and certainly will be again, "down."

Meet Jim Martin

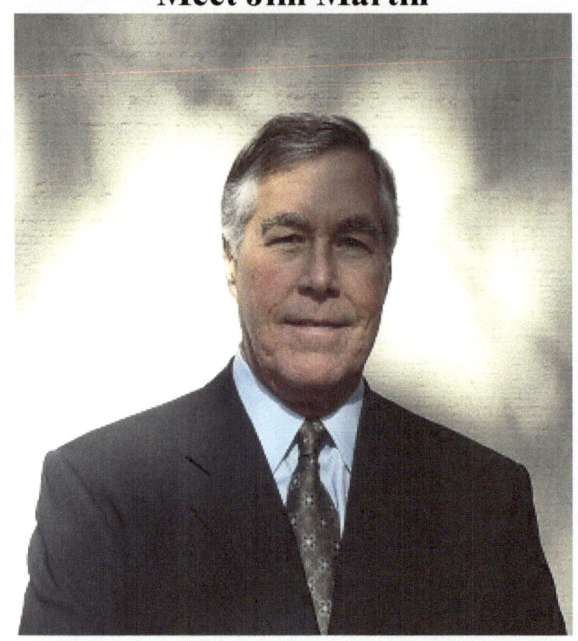

After 30 years practicing law as a trial attorney primarily representing physicians in medical malpractice litigation, Jim is a brain injury survivor whose career ended in December, 2010 when he experienced a significant traumatic brain injury, and resulting permanent memory impairment.

Following an extended period of time learning to accept his new reality, he now volunteers with the Alzheimer's Association, where he is a Board member, attends support group meetings with Brain Injury Connections NW, is a member of Brain Injury Alliance of Oregon, and volunteers at a local Portland, Oregon hospital.

To stay connected with the legal community, Jim mentors newly admitted lawyers with the Oregon State Bar.

Yesterday is not ours to recover, but tomorrow is ours to win or lose.

— Lyndon B. Johnson

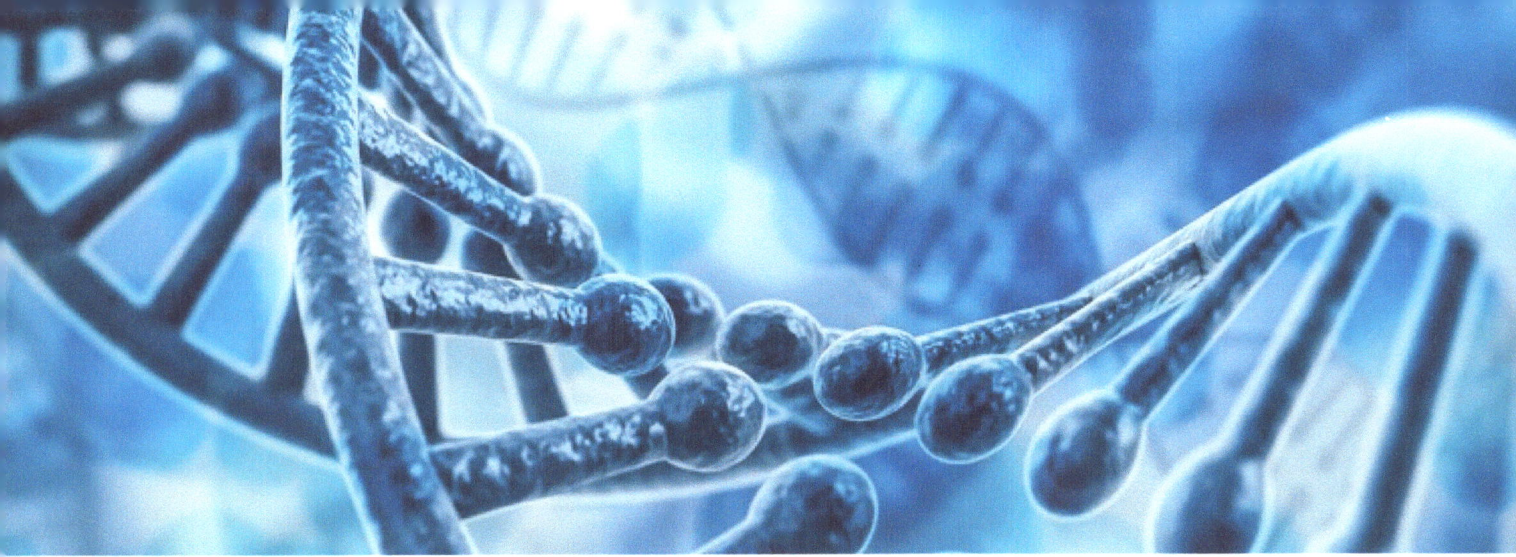

The Evolution of Life

By David A. Grant

Early on, during the first few years after my brain injury, it seemed like we lived and breathed "all things TBI." Not a day went by when the conversation didn't drift to traumatic brain injury. Sometimes it was a passing comment, while at other times, it became the focal point of our day.

In all fairness, how could it not? Years ago I heard that brain injury is the last thing you think about – until it's the only thing you think about. My brain injury was singularly the biggest game-changer of our lives. If affected me, my wife Sarah, my mom and dad, my children, and my stepchildren. If you knew me before my accident, you were in some way affected. Such is the all-inclusive nature of a traumatic brain injury.

But time passes, as it inevitably does. And those three words that we hear all the time come to pass: Life Goes On.

I could fill a book or two about all that has happened since that fated day back in 2010. Next week marks the six year anniversary of my cycling accident. It was on a sunny late-Fall day in November of 2010 that life as we knew it ended abruptly in a twisted mess of broken steel and shattered glass.

Today I have something that I didn't have early on. I now have the benefit of perspective as I can look back through many years of a post-trauma life. And through that prism of perspective, I can see how much we have evolved.

No longer is brain injury the centerpiece of our lives. Don't get me wrong. There isn't a day that goes by that it doesn't rear its head. Trouble finding a word? Overwhelming day-ending exhaustion by 3:00 PM, forgetting something rather important – then promptly forgetting it again (and perhaps a third time for good measure.)

TBI reminds us that life will never be the same.

But on many days, brain injury does not ride shotgun—it is relegated to the back seat. You know that it's there, but its presence is secondary. I can't begin to tell you how good that feels.

There is a rhythm, an ebb and flow to most days that is relatively predictable. During the week, Sarah and I roll out of bed early. Some days she heads to her office, other days she works from home. I roll into my office by 8:00 AM after breakfast, coffee, and a few minutes of morning news. I work diligently until lunchtime. If it's a day that Sarah is working from home, we head out for a quick lunch together; then it's back to my desk for a while.

Most every afternoon, I take my cycling break – trekking twenty-five miles or so on my bike through the back roads of southern New Hampshire. Cycling has done more to help me recover than just about anything.

A healthy body helps speed the healing process of a damaged brain. Science long ago proved this. Our nights can be pretty full as well. Gone are the days when I was rendered useless by my injury.

Most days are just like that – average, uneventful days packed full of life.

Having a brain injury means that I have a lifelong condition. The evolution of life after brain injury does indeed go on. Early on, there were no good days, just good moments.

As time passed, there was an occasional good day, but most were still dark and foreboding. Life is such that now, most days are pretty average.

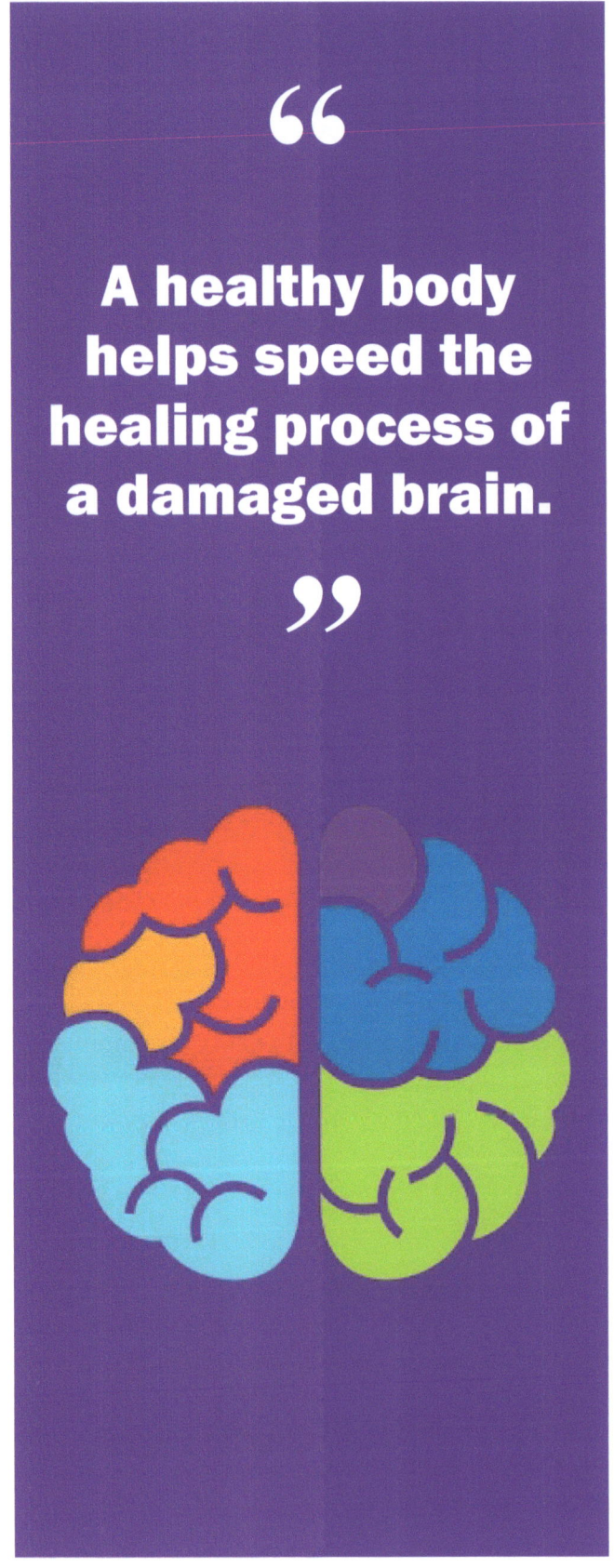

A healthy body helps speed the healing process of a damaged brain.

Occasionally I have a really good day, and occasionally I have a really abysmal day. The takeaway is this: I can see progress. I am not who I was before my accident. That guy died in 2010. But I am also not who I was in early recovery. I am slowly healing along with my wife, Sarah, and our family. We are learning to coexist with the elephant in the living room.

Taking this one step further, in a few years, I will not be who I am today, as the healing will continue. Looking at how far we have come, it's hard not to be excited about that.

Meet David A. Grant

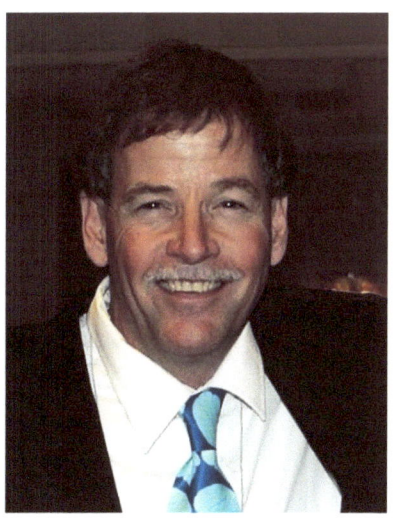

David A. Grant is a freelance writer based out of southern New Hampshire and the publisher of TBI HOPE Magazine. He is the author of Metamorphosis, Surviving Brain Injury.

He is also a contributing author to Chicken Soup for the Soul, Recovering from Traumatic Brain Injuries. David is a BIANH Board Member as well as a member of the Brain Energy Support Team Board of Directors.

David is a regular contributing writer to Brainline.org, a PBS sponsored website.

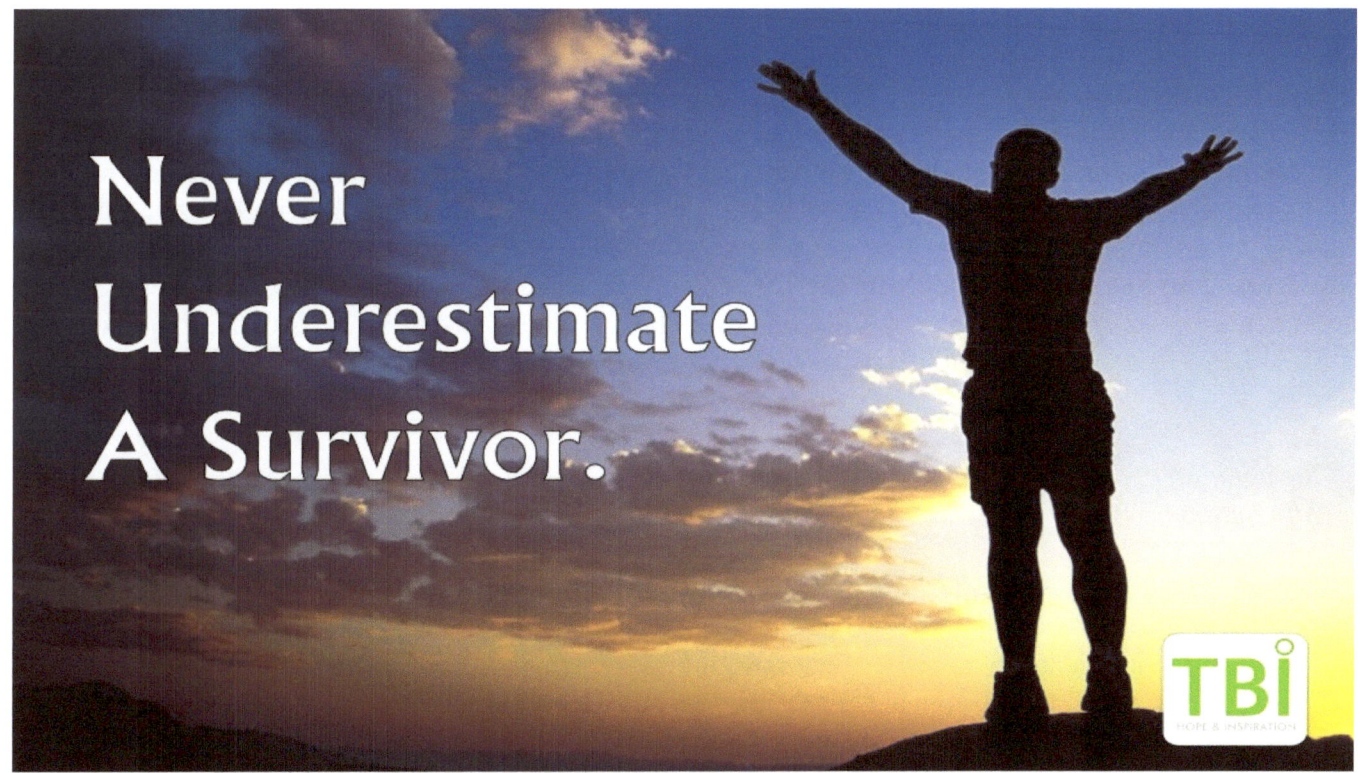

Never Underestimate A Survivor.

TBI

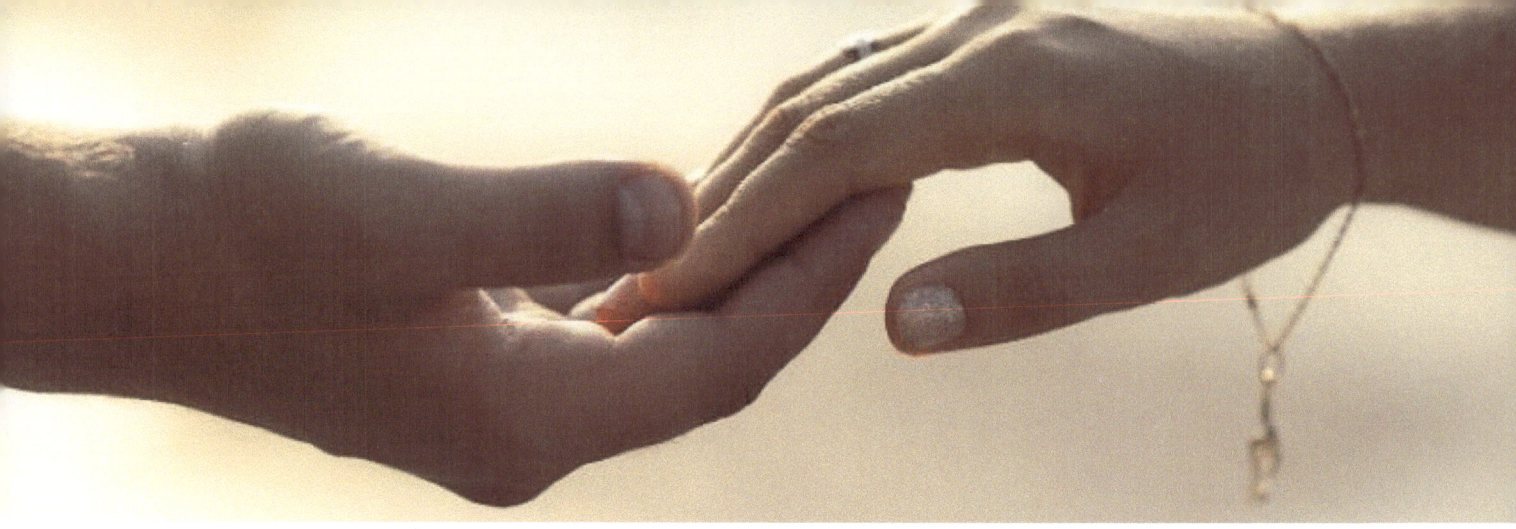

Five Skills for the Resilient Caregiver
By Janet M. Cromer, RN, MA, LMHC

A Caregiver is a Partner.

That's true for both the survivor and caregiver or care partner. Whether you are a new caregiver or a seasoned pro, there are five foundation skills that can enhance your health and resilience: 1) Embrace self-compassion. 2) Counterbalance the stress response. 3) Live mindfully. 4) Construct sustaining connections. 5) Express your creativity. Studies have shown that cultivating these skills, and others, can help reduce the risk of burnout and compassion fatigue. Self-compassion is the gateway skill because it empowers us to prioritize self-care. Carlos cares for his wife who has a brain tumor. He showers Maria with compassion and kindness while encouraging her to talk and feed herself. He criticizes himself harshly for not being able to take away her sorrow or pain. He imagines a caregiving judge holding up a low score card, like the mean judges on the TV dancing shows he watches. So, how can a caregiver shift from neglect to self-compassion? Dr. Kristen Neff, in her book Self-Compassion: Stop Beating Yourself Up and Leave Insecurity Behind, describes self-compassion as having three components:

> *Kindness*
> *Recognition of our common humanity*
> *Mindfulness*

Kindness means that we actively soothe and empathize with ourselves, much as we would with a friend who is going through a rough time. One of the most healing changes to make is to replace your inner critic with an inner mentor to guide you on your journey. You can visualize an inner mentor by remembering a trusted friend, colleague, or family member in whom you could confide. Imagine that person's presence and voice as he or she listens and responds to you with compassion and wisdom. Carlos visualized his Uncle Alfred smiling warmly as he said, "Ah, Carlos. You show Maria so much love. You're a top-scoring husband! Relax and enjoy your time together." Self-compassion heightens self-respect. One way this might manifest is in setting healthy boundaries. Have a conversation with the person you care for about how you plan to show each other respect through your communication and behavior. Another core component of self-compassion is our shared humanity. This means that you take pride in all that you contribute to the person you care for and others. You take responsibility for what you can, but also forgive your mistakes. It's a relief to realize that we are only human, with the talents and limitations that implies!

Reverse the Stress Response

The second foundation skill is to counterbalance the stress response. The stress response evolved as a brilliant survival mechanism meant to give you the power to fight off a threat or run for your life. This response starts automatically, whether the perceived threat is physical or emotional, real or imagined. The chemical and hormonal activation that the body and mind undergo is meant to subside within a few hours after the danger ends. Contrast a few hours with the weeks or months of unremitting stress that some caregivers experience. That may be one reason caregivers have higher rates of chronic illness than non-caregivers. First, learn to identify your personal stress triggers and signals. What sets you off? How do your body and mind react? Margaret said, "When I have to argue with my husband to take his blood pressure pills, my whole back knots up and I want to scream at him." Her husband always likes dessert, so Margaret decided to quietly offer him the pills before serving the cake. Awareness empowers you to intervene early. Think of ways to prevent or minimize how often your trigger happens. Learning ways to elicit a more relaxed state of being pays off in health dividends. Proven techniques include meditation, mindfulness, yoga, tai chi, time in nature, and repetitive exercise such as swimming laps. Schedule daily respite breaks, and do whatever it takes to get away regularly.

Take the Mystery out of Mindfulness

The third foundation skill is to live mindfully. Does this mean that you have to withdraw from the world and meditate for hours a day? Not at all! Mindfulness means being in the present moment as fully as possible without judging or exaggerating your feelings or experiences. It means being aware of both the good and the difficult, and being open to new approaches. There are many forms of mindfulness meditation. You can find classes, books, and CDs to guide your practice. Sitting quietly and focusing on the flow of your breath is an effective way to start. Early in the morning, set a positive intention for your day. Build in "peak moments" of small sensory or emotional pleasures and give them your full attention.

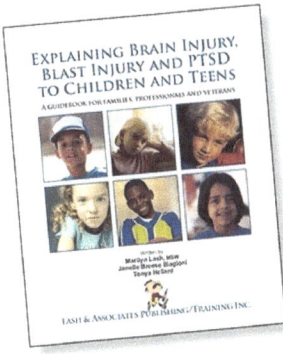

Carlos bit into a ripe peach and savored the fragrance and juice. Throughout the day, do a body scan to release tension and attend to a hidden emotion. At the end of the day, list three things that you did well.

Construct Connections

The fourth foundation skill is to build sustaining connections. Avoid the isolation that can trap caregivers and contribute to stress and compassion fatigue. Think about what you need from friends and helpers at this juncture, and what you can contribute to a relationship. Be honest. Then train people in how to help you. Do you want someone to listen while you vent, or help you problem solve? Margaret asked a young neighbor to look up information on the Internet for her. Cultivate relationships with people who share your experiences, as well as those with a different perspective who can help you grow. Call on a professional counselor to heal trauma, explore intense emotions, or learn adjustment skills. One of the advantages of trusting supporters is that we are less likely to keep dangerous secrets. Brain injury caregivers can witness, or be the target of verbal outbursts, substance abuse, or physical aggression. Sometimes we hide these problems out of fear or shame, but the first priority must be to keep everyone in the family safe.

Express Yourself

Expressing your creativity in as many ways as possible is the fifth foundation skill. You might write a journal or blog, draw or paint, or tell your story to raise awareness. Creativity invites you to claim ownership of your narrative, integrate emotions, and gain a new perspective. Getting absorbed in a hobby or fun activity is a proven stress buster! Carlos noticed that when he strummed his guitar and sang, he felt at peace instead of worrying. Whether you paint a landscape, cook up a pot of chili, or build a bookcase, you're in control of the process and the outcome. You have something to show for your time, and you get better at that skill.

Meet Janet M. Cromer

Janet Cromer, RN, MA, LMHC is a psychiatric RN and the author of "Professor Cromer Learns to Read: A Couple's New Life after Brain Injury."

Janet speaks nationally on family and professional caregiver issues including stress resilience, traumatic stress, compassion renewal, seasons of caregiving, and creativity and healing. See more at www.janetcromer.com.

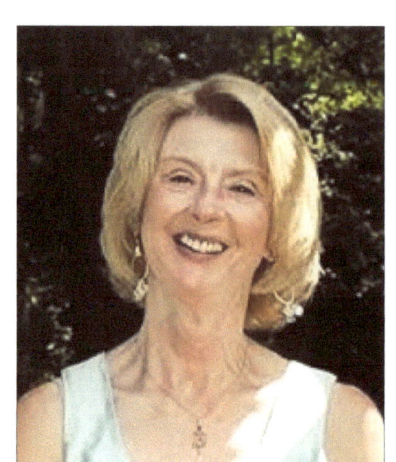

THE BACKPAGE

You've just read about some amazing people who have found a way to live meaningful lives after brain injury. Jen and Donna, Rosalie, Derek, James, Melissa and Barbara, and Amy. These are not just names in print, they are all people who live with something they never asked for and never expected.

Their courage in the sharing of their stories will touch the lives of others, acting as a beacon of hope in the often dark and confusing world of brain injury.

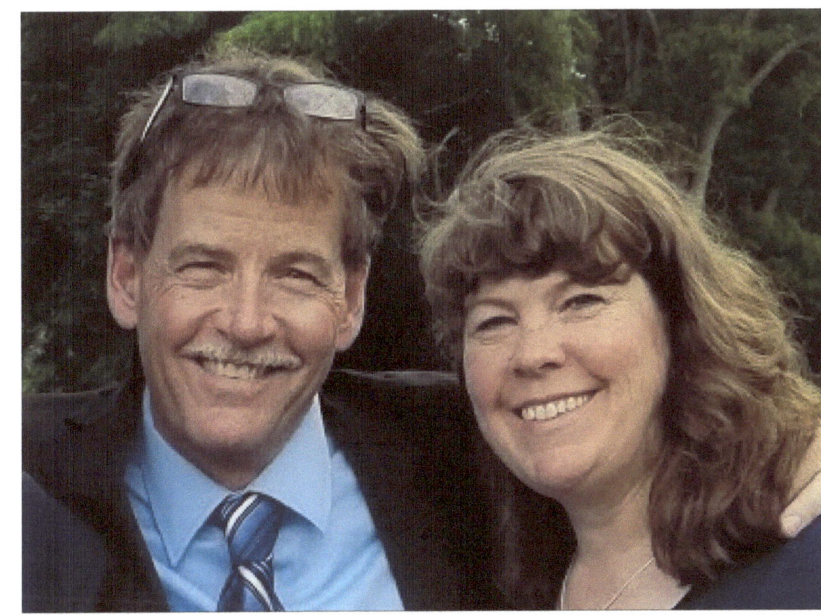

We all have something to offer to others, to help lift humanity higher. Your offering need not be large, or even in the public eye.

Holding the door for a stranger who needs assistance, a kind word to someone having a bad day, an email to a friend letting them know they are in your thoughts… none of these simple tasks takes much time but they can change the course of someone's entire day.

Kindness is indeed catchy.

We encourage you to reflect on your life, and if the opportunity presents itself, to give of yourself in some small way. I'll let you in on a little secret: when you give of yourself to others, you change as well.

My wife Sarah and I live lives we never envisioned. There are still very tough days. That goes with our lives as a survivor family. But there are times, times like this, when we reflect on the people that are now part of the fabric of our lives, that we realize that we are truly blessed beyond measure.

May you find peace in your journey,

~David & Sarah

www.ingramcontent.com/pod-product-compliance
Lightning Source LLC
Chambersburg PA
CBHW060808290526
45792CB00005BA/1563